PMH-BC™ Certification Practice Q&A

PMH-BC™ Certification Practice Q&A

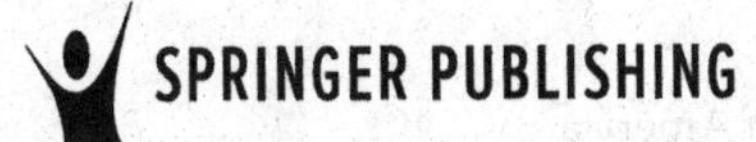

Springer Publishing Company, LLC
11 West 42nd Street, New York, NY 10036
www.springerpub.com

Acquisitions Editor: Elizabeth Nieginski
Compositor: diacriTech

ISBN: 9780826146120
ebook ISBN: 9780826146137
DOI: 10.1891/9780826146137

Printed by BnT

Medicine is an ever-changing science. Research and clinical experience are continually expanding our knowledge , in particular our understanding of proper treatment and drug therapy. The authors, editors, and publisher have made every effort to ensure that all information in this book is in accordance with the state of knowledge at the time of production of the book. Nevertheless, the authors, editors, and publisher are not responsible for any errors or omissions or for any consequence from application of the information in this book and make no warranty, expressed or implied, with respect to the content of this publication. Every reader should examine carefully the package inserts accompanying each drug and should carefully check whether the dosage schedules therein or the contraindications stated by the manufacturer differ from the statements made in this book. Such examination is particularly important with drugs that are either rarely used or have been newly released on the market. The publisher has no responsibility for the persistence or accuracy of URLs for external or third-party Internet websites referred to in this publication and does not guarantee that any content on such websites is, or will remain, accurate or appropriate.

LCCN: 2022942173

Contact sales@springerpub.com to receive discount rates on bulk purchases.

Publisher's Note: **New and used products purchased from third-party sellers are not guaranteed for quality, authenticity, or access to any included digital components.**

PMH-BC™ is a registered trademark of American Nurses Credentialing Center (ANCC®). ANCC® does not sponsor or endorse this resource, nor does it have a proprietary relationship with Springer Publishing.

Printed in the United States of America.

Contents

Preface

Welcome to *PMH-BC™ Certification Practice Q&A*! Congratulations on taking this important step on your journey to becoming a certified psychiatric–mental health nurse. This resource is based on the most recent Psychiatric-Mental Health Nursing Certification (PMH-BC™) exam blueprint and was developed by experienced psychiatric–mental health nurses. It is designed to help you sharpen your specialty knowledge with 150 practice questions organized by exam subject area, as well as strengthen your knowledge-application and test-taking skills with a 150-question practice exam. It also includes essential information about the PMH-BC™ exam, including eligibility requirements, exam subject areas and question distribution, and tips for successful exam preparation.

PART I: PRACTICE QUESTIONS

Part I includes four chapters based on the exam blueprint: Assessment and Diagnosis, Planning, Implementation, and Evaluation. Each chapter includes high-quality, exam-style questions and comprehensive answers with rationales that address both correct and incorrect answers. Part I is designed to strengthen your specialty knowledge and is formatted for ultimate studying convenience—answer the questions on each page and simply turn the page for the corresponding answers and rationales. No need to refer to the back of the book for the answers.

PART II: PRACTICE EXAMINATION

Part II includes a 150-question practice exam that aligns with the content domains and question distribution on the most recent PMH-BC™ exam blueprint. This practice exam is designed to help you strengthen your knowledge-application and test-taking skills. Maximize your preparation and simulate the exam experience by setting aside 3 hours to complete the practice exam. Comprehensive answers and rationales that address both correct and incorrect answers are located in the chapter immediately following the practice exam.

We know life is busy, and being able to prepare for your exam efficiently and effectively is paramount. This resource will give you the tools and confidence you need to succeed. For additional exam preparation resources, including self-paced online courses, online QBanks, comprehensive review texts, and high-yield study guides, visit www.springerpub.com/examprep. Best of luck to you on your certification journey!

Introduction: PMH-BC™ Certification Exam and Tips for Preparation

▶ ELIGIBILITY REQUIREMENTS

The Psychiatric-Mental Health Nursing Certification (PMH-BC™) exam is developed and administered by the American Nurses Credentialing Center (ANCC). To qualify to take the exam, you must meet the following requirements:

- Hold a current, active RN license in a state or territory of the United States or hold the professional, legally recognized equivalent in another country.
- Have practiced the equivalent of 2 years full-time as a registered nurse.
- Have a minimum of 2,000 hours of clinical practice in psychiatric–mental health nursing within the past 3 years.
- Have completed 30 hours of continuing education in psychiatric–mental health nursing within the past 3 years.

Qualified applicants may submit an online application. Successful candidates will receive an Authorization to Test and can self-schedule their exam. The exam fee is $395; discounted fees are available for members of the American Nurses Association ($295), the American Psychiatric Nurses Association ($220), and the International Society of Psychiatric-Mental Health Nurses ($340). Refer to the ANCC website for complete eligibility requirements, pricing, and certification information: https://www.nursingworld.org/our-certifications/psychiatric-mental-health-nursing-certification/

▶ ABOUT THE EXAMINATION

The PMH-BC™ exam takes 3 hours and consists of 150 multiple-choice questions with four answer options. You must select the single best answer. Only 150 questions are scored, and the remaining 25 questions are used as pretest questions. It is impossible to know which questions are scored, so be sure to answer all questions to the best of your ability.

See Table 1 for exam content domains and question distribution. For more detailed exam content information, refer to the PMH-BC™ Test Content Outline at https://www.nursingworld.org/~49969b/globalassets/certification/certification-specialty-pages/resources/test-content-outlines/psychnurse-tco-after.pdf.

Table 1. PMH-BC™ Exam Content Domains and Question Distribution

Content Domain	Percentage of Questions
Assessment and diagnosis	22%
Planning	22%
Implementation	39%
Evaluation	18%

TIPS FOR EXAM PREPARATION

You know the old joke about how to get to Carnegie Hall—practice, practice, practice! The same is true when seeking certification. Practice and preparation are key to your success on exam day. Here are 10 tips to help you prepare:

1. Allow at least 6 months to fully prepare for the exam. Do not rely on last-minute cramming sessions.
2. Thoroughly review the PMH-BC™ Test Content Outline so that you know exactly what to expect. Pay close attention to the content domains, subdomains, and topics. Identify your strengths, weaknesses, and knowledge gaps, so you know where to focus your studies. Review all of the supplementary resources available on the ANCC website.
3. Create a study timeline with weekly or monthly study tasks. Be as specific as possible—identify *what* you will study, *how* you will study, and *when* you will study.
4. Use several examination preperation resources that provide different benefits. For example, use a comprehensive review to build your specialty knowledge, use this resource and other question banks to strengthen your knowledge-application and test-taking skills, and use a high-yield review to brush up on key concepts in the days leading up to the exam. Springer Publishing offers a wide range of print and online exam prep products to suit all of your study needs; visit https://www.springerpub.com/examprep.
5. Assess your level of knowledge and performance on practice questions and exams. Carefully consider why you may be missing certain questions. Continually analyze your strengths, weaknesses, and knowledge gaps, and adjust your study plan accordingly.
6. Minimize distraction as much as possible while you are studying. You will feel more calm, centered, and focused, which will lead to increased knowledge retention.
7. Engage in stress-reducing activities, particularly in the month leading up to the exam. Yoga, stretching, and deep-breathing exercises can be beneficial. If you are feeling frustrated or anxious while studying, take a break. Go for a walk, play with your child or pet, or finish a chore that has been weighing on you. Wait until you feel more refreshed before returning to study.

8. Focus on your health in the weeks and days before the exam. Eat balanced meals, stay hydrated, and minimize alcohol consumption. Get as much sleep as possible, particularly the night before the examination.
9. Eat a light meal before the exam but limit your liquid consumption. The clock does not stop for restroom breaks! Ensure that you know exactly where you are going and how long it will take to get there. Leave with plenty of time to spare to reduce travel-related stress and ensure that you arrive on time.
10. Remind yourself to relax and stay calm. You have prepared, and you know your stuff. Visualize the success that is just ahead of you and make it happen. When you pass, celebrate!

Pass Guarantee

If you use this resource to prepare for your exam and do not pass, you may return it for a refund of your full purchase price, excluding tax, shipping, and handling. To receive a refund, return your product along with a copy of your exam score report and original receipt showing purchase of new product (not used). Product must be returned and received within 180 days of the original purchase date. Refunds will be issued within 8 weeks from acceptance and approval. One offer per person and address. This offer is valid for U.S. residents only. Void where prohibited. To initiate a refund, please contact Customer Service at csexamprep@springerpub.com.

Part I

Practice Questions and Answers With Rationales

Assessment and Diagnosis

1. The nurse reviews the health record of a new patient diagnosed with major depressive disorder and documented psychomotor agitation. The nurse should expect to observe:

   A. Hypersomnia, leaden paralysis, or significant weight gain/increased appetite
   B. Rubbing or pulling of the skin, difficulty sitting still, or wringing of hands
   C. Difficulty controlling worry, muscle tension, and irritability
   D. Repetitive handwashing, counting, or repeating words silently

2. The nurse is reviewing autopsy results for a 70-year-old patient with Alzheimer disease. The report notes that the brain has diffuse atrophy with flattened cortical sulci and enlarged ventricles. Microscopic examination of the brain most likely shows decreased:

   A. Dopamine
   B. Acetylcholine
   C. Serotonin
   D. Tryptophan

3. The nurse is reviewing the chart of a 7-year-old patient and notes that genetic testing reveals an extra chromosome 21, which indicates:

   A. Down syndrome
   B. Rett syndrome
   C. Fragile X syndrome
   D. Prader–Willi syndrome

4. To assess for normal behavioral development of a 3-year-old, the nurse asks the toddler to perform a task such as:

   A. Building a tower of nine cubes
   B. Skipping using feet alternately
   C. Standing on one foot for 5 seconds
   D. Tying their shoelaces

(See answers next page.)

1. B) Rubbing or pulling of the skin, difficulty sitting still, or wringing of hands

Rubbing or pulling of skin, difficulty sitting still, and wringing hands are all examples of psychomotor agitation. Hypersomnia, leaden paralysis, and significant weight gain/increased appetite are examples of atypical features of depression. Difficulty controlling worry, muscle tension, and irritability together are features of generalized anxiety disorder. Repetitive handwashing, counting, and repeating words silently are compulsions that can occur in patients with obsessive-compulsive disorder.

2. B) Acetylcholine

Acetylcholine is associated with attention and memory and is decreased in Alzheimer disease. The medications used to help manage Alzheimer disease are acetylcholinesterase inhibitors, which help to reduce the breakdown of acetylcholine. Dopamine is also involved with thinking but is implicated in Parkinson disease, in which dopamine is decreased. Serotonin is associated with regulation of sleep and mood; it is most implicated as being decreased in depression and anxiety. Tryptophan is not a neurotransmitter, but an amino acid and a precursor to serotonin.

3. A) Down syndrome

Down syndrome, or trisomy 21, is caused by an extra copy of chromosome 21. Rett syndrome is caused by a dominant X-linked gene mutation. Inactivation of the *FMR-1* gene is seen in fragile X syndrome, and Prader–Willi syndrome is a deletion in chromosome 15q12.

4. A) Building a tower of nine cubes

A 3-year-old is able to build a tower of 9 to 10 cubes, copy a circle and a cross, ride a tricycle, jump from the bottom step, alternate feet going up stairs, put on their shoes, unbutton buttons, and feed themself. A 5-year-old can skip using feet alternately, a 4-year-old can stand on one foot for 5 to 8 seconds, and a 6-year-old can tie their shoelaces.

5. The nurse is performing a physical assessment on a child who is able to print their name, tie their shoelaces, and count 10 objects accurately. These developmental milestones would indicate that the child is how many years old?

A. 3
B. 4
C. 5
D. 6

6. The nurse is assessing a 6-year-old patient who is cognitively impaired, makes poor eye contact, and does not interact socially with peers. The patient was born with spina bifida that required surgery. The patient's mother reports taking medications for a seizure disorder and depression while pregnant. The medication the nurse suspects the patient's mother was taking during pregnancy is:

A. Folate
B. Paroxetine
C. Lamotrigine
D. Valproate

7. The nurse is evaluating an older adult patient. In the mental state examination, the nurse asks the patient to interpret proverbs. The patient's responses are literal. The nurse notes that the patient has a pattern of concrete interpretation. This indicates:

A. Poor insight
B. Poor judgment
C. Delusional thought content
D. Deficit in cognitive thinking

8. The nurse is evaluating a patient who reports that they are sad. The nurse documents this finding as:

A. Thought content
B. Thought process
C. Patient affect
D. Patient mood

(See answers next page.)

5. D) 6

By 6 years old, a child should be able to ride a two-wheel bicycle, count 10 objects correctly, print their name, copy a triangle, and tie shoelaces. A 3-year-old is able to build a tower of 9 to 10 cubes, copy a circle and a cross, ride a tricycle, jump from a bottom step, alternate feet going upstairs, put on their shoes, unbutton buttons, and feed themself. A 4-year-old can walk downstairs one step at a time, stand on one foot for 5 to 8 seconds, copy a cross, repeat four digits, count three objects correctly, brush their own teeth, and wash and dry their face. A 5-year-old will skip using feet alternately, have complete sphincter control, copy a square, dress and undress themself, and print a few letters.

6. D) Valproate

Valproate is associated with with neural tube defects, such as spina bifida. Furthermore, valproate is associated with cognitive decline in school-age children, and it may increase the risk of autism spectrum disorder. Folate, given in supplements as folic acid, is used to protect the neural development of a fetus, and all pregnant patients should be instructed to take folic acid. Although paroxetine is a teratogen, it does not cause neural tube defects, but is associated with cardiac malformations. Lamotrigine is associated with cleft palate.

7. D) Deficit in cognitive thinking

Abstraction requires higher cognitive or intellectual functioning. Abstract reasoning is the ability to shift back and forth between general concepts and specific examples. The inability to think abstractly indicates concrete or literal thinking. This may be seen in an older adult as a sign of early dementia. Insight refers to the patient's understanding of how they feel. Judgment refers to the patient's capacity to make good decisions and act on them. Delusional thought content refers to false beliefs not shared by others.

8. D) Patient mood

Mood is defined as the patient's internal and sustained emotional state. It is a subjective report of what the patient states they feel. Affect differs from mood in that it is the expression of mood that is reflected in the patient's appearance and what the nurse observes. Thought content is what type of thoughts are occurring to the patient, which are described during the context of the evaluation. Thought process differs from thought content because it describes how thoughts are formulated rather than what a person is thinking.

9. The nurse is evaluating a patient who expresses delusional thoughts that are grandiose in nature. The nurse documents this finding as:

A. Thought process
B. Thought content
C. Patient mood
D. Patient affect

10. The psychiatric–mental health nurse is evaluating a patient who has flight of ideas. This is documented in the mental state examination as:

A. Thought content
B. Thought process
C. Patient mood
D. Patient affect

11. A patient presenting with severe hyperthermia, muscle rigidity, diaphoresis, and ocular clonus reports having taken an overdose of a prescribed psychiatric medication approximately 12 hours ago. The nurse suspects an overdose of:

A. Benzodiazepine
B. Serotonin and norepinephrine reuptake inhibitor (SNRI) anticholinergic
C. Monoamine oxidase inhibitor (MAOI)
D. Tricyclic antidepressant (TCA)

(See answers next page.)

9. B) Thought content

Thought content describes what type of thoughts are occurring to the patient, which are described during the context of the evaluation. These can be obsessional, suicidal, homicidal, or delusional thoughts. Thought process differs from thought content because it describes how thoughts are formulated rather than what the person is thinking. Affect is the expression of mood that is reflected in the patient's appearance and what the nurse observes. Mood refers to the patient's internal and sustained emotional state; it is a subjective report of what the patient states they feel.

10. B) Thought process

Thought process describes how thoughts are formulated, organized, and expressed. A patient can have normal thought process with delusional thought content, or normal thought content with impaired thought process. Normal thought process is described as organized, linear, and goal directed. Impaired thought process can be described as flight of ideas, circumstantiality, clang association, derailment, neologism, perseveration, tangentiality, or thought blocking. Thought content differs from thought process because it describes what types of thoughts are occurring to the patient, which are described during the context of the evaluation. Affect is the expression of mood that is reflected in the patient's appearance and what the nurse observes. Mood refers to the patient's internal and sustained emotional state; it is a subjective report of what the patient states they feel.

11. C) Monoamine oxidase inhibitor (MAOI)

Signs and symptoms of MAOI overdose range from mild to severe. Severe symptoms include severe hyperthermia, seizures, central nervous system depression, muscle rigidity, and myoclonus. Clinical features of acute intoxication with a benzodiazepine include slurred speech, incoordination (ataxia), unsteady gait, and impaired attention or memory; physical signs include nystagmus and decreased reflexes. Anticholinergic syndrome presents with flushing, dry mucous membranes and skin, fever, and altered mental state. TCAs are common agents used in cases of fatal overdose, with signs and symptoms that include fever, drowsiness, confusion, and cardiac arrest.

12. The nurse is assessing a 7-year-old patient with reports of decreased concentration, hyperactivity, short attention span, and being easily distracted. The patient's parent reports that the child is not able to complete simple tasks at home, such as bed making, and does not complete homework. More information is needed, so a screening tool is sent home with the patient's parent, including one for the patient's teacher, to be filled out and brought back to the next visit. The screening tool being used is the:

A. Young Mania Rating Scale
B. Conners Rating Scale
C. Hamilton Anxiety Rating Scale
D. Brief Psychiatric Rating Scale

13. A clinician-rated scale that is used to assess a patient's anxiety symptoms is the:

A. GAD-7
B. CAPS
C. PHQ-9
D. HAM-A

14. A patient presents for evaluation of post-traumatic stress disorder (PTSD). The tool that would be used to assess the severity of the patient's symptoms is:

A. CAPS
B. PDSS
C. HAM-A
D. HAM-D

15. A patient is suspected to have a cognitive disorder. The assessment tool used to further assess the patient's cognition is the:

A. BDI
B. HAM-D
C. HAM-A
D. MMSE

(See answers next page.)

12. B) Conners Rating Scale

The patient is exhibiting signs and symptoms of attention deficit hyperactivity disorder (ADHD). The Conners Rating Scale is used to help clinicians measure a range of childhood mental health disorders and is used most commonly to screen for ADHD symptoms. The Conners Rating Scale has parent, teacher, and self-report versions. The Young Mania Rating Scale is used to screen for bipolar disorder, the Hamilton Anxiety Rating Scale is used to screen for anxiety, and the Brief Psychiatric Rating Scale is used to assess for change or improvement in psychotic patients. Although it is important to screen for all possible mental health disorders, the Conners Rating Scale is the only scale that has both parent and teacher rating components; the other scales are clinician-administered screening tools.

13. D) HAM-A

The Hamilton Anxiety Rating Scale (HAM-A) is a 14-item clinician-rated anxiety scale used to assess both cognitive and somatic anxiety symptoms. A score of 14 is the threshold for clinically significant anxiety. The GAD-7, or Generalized Anxiety Disorder 7-item Questionnaire, examines a patient's self-reported symptoms of anxiety. The CAPS, or Clinician-Administered PTSD Scale, is a 17-item scale used specifically to assess for post-traumatic stress disorder. The PHQ-9, or Patient Health Questionnaire–9, is a nine-item patient-reported screening tool for symptoms of depression.

14. A) CAPS

The CAPS, or Clinician-Administered PTSD Scale, is a 17-item scale that clinicians use to diagnose PTSD. The items can also be used to generate a total PTSD severity score, which is obtained by adding the frequency and intensity scales for each item. The PDSS is the Panic Disorder Severity Scale, which can be useful in determining severity of panic attacks; these may or may not be present in someone with PTSD. The HAM-A, or Hamilton Anxiety Rating Scale, is used to assess for generalized anxiety disorder, which may be comorbid with PTSD. However, it does not measure PTSD symptom severity. The HAM-D, or Hamilton Rating Scale for Depression, is used to assess for major depression in patients, which too may be comorbid in some patients with PTSD; however, the HAM-D does not measure PTSD symptom severity.

15. D) MMSE

The MMSE, or Mini-Mental State Examination, is a 30-point cognitive test that is used to assess a broad array of cognitive functions, including attention, memory, cognition, and construction of language. The Beck Depression Inventory (BDI) and Hamilton Rating Scale for Depression (HAM-D) would both be useful if the nurse suspects an underlying depressive symptomology that could co-occur or mimic a cognitive disorder. The HAM-A, or Hamilton Anxiety Rating Scale, would be useful in evaluating a patient who is suspected of having an anxiety disorder.

16. The nurse is screening a patient for alcohol use disorder using the CAGE questionnaire. To assess the "A" in CAGE, the nurse asks:

    A. "Have you felt anxious about your drinking?"
    B. "Have people felt alarmed by your drinking?"
    C. "Have people annoyed you by criticizing your drinking?"
    D. "Have you felt that you needed to drink to feel awake?"

17. The nurse is working in the psychiatric emergency department and wants to quickly screen a patient suspected of alcohol use disorder. The screening tool that best meets the needs of the nurse is the:

    A. CAGE questionnaire
    B. MAST screening
    C. ASI measure
    D. PDSS

18. The nurse is assessing a 3-year-old child who has short palpebral fissures, a smooth philtrum with a thin upper lip, and some learning disabilities. The nurse would assess for a central nervous system (CNS) manifestation of:

    A. Microphthalmia
    B. Midface hypoplasia
    C. Microcephaly
    D. Growth restriction

(See answers next page.)

16. C) "Have people annoyed you by criticizing your drinking?"
The CAGE questionnaire is a brief screening tool to assess for significant alcohol problems. CAGE is an acronym used to guide the clinician in their questioning, as follows: C: Have you ever felt you needed to cut down on your drinking? A: Have people annoyed you by criticizing your drinking? G: Have you ever felt guilty or bad about your drinking? E: Have you ever had a drink first thing in the morning to get rid of a hangover (eye-opener)? Each yes answer is scored as 1 point, for a total of 4 points. A score of 1 needs further evaluation, and a score of 2 or more indicates significant alcohol problems.

17. A) CAGE questionnaire
The CAGE questionnaire is a quick screening tool for significant alcohol problems. CAGE is an acronym used to guide the clinician in their questioning, as follows: C: Have you ever felt you needed to cut down on your drinking? A: Have people annoyed you by criticizing your drinking? G: Have you ever felt guilty or bad about your drinking? E: Have you ever had a drink first thing in the morning to get rid of a hangover (eye-opener)? Each yes answer is scored as 1 point for a total of 4 points. A score of 1 needs further evaluation, and a score of 2 or more indicates significant alcohol problems. The Michigan Alcoholism Screening Test (MAST) is a 22-item self-report. The ASI, or Addiction Severity Index, measures of symptoms, is a comprehensive quantitative tool used by clinicians to assess alcohol or drug disorders; it takes more than 1 hour in a structured interview to perform. The PDSS, or Panic Disorder Severity Scale, is used to screen for panic disorder, not alcohol use disorder.

18. C) Microcephaly
The nurse would assess for the CNS manifestation of microcephaly. The sequelae that this child presents with is seen in fetal alcohol syndrome. The characteristics of fetal alcohol syndrome include growth restriction, microphthalmia, midface hypoplasia, short palpebral fissures, a smooth philtrum, and a thin upper lip. The CNS manifestations include microcephaly, attention deficits, hyperactivity, and a history of delayed development with learning disabilities and even seizures.

19. The nurse is evaluating a 13-year-old patient. The parent states, "He has tantrums like a 6-year-old. When he is not having tantrums, he is just angry at the world. He's lost most of his friends. He has been like this for the past 2 years, and it is just getting worse." To gather additional information to support the suspected diagnosis, the nurse asks:

A. "Have your child's mood problems been episodic?"
B. "Has your child ever shown physical aggression toward animals?"
C. "Has there been any suspected abuse of your child?"
D. "Are there any difficulties with distraction or hyperactivity?"

20. A patient has recently given birth and reports feelings of low mood, tearfulness, and inability to sleep due to worrying about the newborn. To help determine if the symptoms are postpartum depression (PPD), the nurse must assess:

A. Time of onset of symptoms
B. Type of patient support system
C. Significant patient weight loss
D. Change in patient appetite

21. After being caught binge drinking on several occasions by their parents, a young adult patient responds to a CAGE screening after presenting to the office. After reviewing the screening, the nurse determines that the patient may be suffering from alcoholism based on the patient saying:

A. "I sometimes drink with my friends, but everyone does it, and it is not a huge deal."
B. "I often feel guilty and think that I need to cut back on how often I drink."
C. "Although I socially drink, I only have one or two drinks a few times a month, if that."
D. "My dad was a functioning alcoholic, so I grew up around it."

(See answers next page.)

19. A) "Have your child's mood problems been episodic?"

The nurse is assessing the patient for disruptive mood dysregulation disorder (DMDD). The clinical presentation is distinctive and involves chronic, non-episodic, and persistent irritability and temper tantrums disproportionate to the trigger. DMDD must be differentiated from bipolar disorder because some of the features of DMDD are similar to those of bipolar disorder. Determining whether the symptom presentation is episodic will help rule out other pathology. Aggression toward animals can be an indicator of abuse; asking about this and about suspected abuse is directed toward investigating trauma-related causes for the patient's behavior. Asking about difficulties with distraction or hyperactivity seeks to rule out the presence of attention deficit hyperactivity disorder. which is not a mood disorder.

20. A) Time of onset of symptoms

Prior to diagnosing a patient with PPD, the nurse must rule out whether the patient is experiencing *baby blues.* Baby blues will occur in 30% to 75% of those who give birth. It can be differentiated from PPD by time of onset and duration. Baby blues typically occur 3 to 5 days after delivery, while PPD occurs within 3 to 6 months after delivery. Duration of baby blues is days to weeks, whereas PPD can last months to years if left untreated. The nurse will also assess type of support system, weight changes, and appetite changes; however, these factors will not differentiate PPD from baby blues.

21. B) "I often feel guilty and think that I need to cut back on how often I drink."

Two elements of the CAGE questionnaire concern whether the patient ever feels the need to "cut back," or whether they ever feel "bad or guilty" about their drinking habits. Having a positive response to two or more of the screening questions may indicate that the person is suffering from alcoholism or alcohol misuse. Occasional social drinking and growing up with a functional alcoholic parent may provide more information about the patient's drinking habits, but an element of the CAGE questionnaire would be needed to determine alcoholism.

22. A teenage patient comes to the office accompanied by their parents for an initial visit. The patient reports worsening symptoms from a traumatic brain injury (TBI) since being involved in a car crash 3 months ago. The nurse suggests that the patient may have a mild neurocognitive disorder due to the TBI. According to the *DSM-5*, this diagnosis involves having one or more symptoms, including:

A. Headaches
B. Poor concentration
C. Amnesia
D. Anxiety

23. An older adult patient comes into the clinic for an initial visit with concerns about worsening symptoms of memory loss over the past 6 months. The provider suspects that the patient may be showing early signs of Alzheimer disease. For an accurate diagnosis, according to the *DSM-5*, the patient must also show signs of:

A. Progressive decline in cognition, with no evidence of any other neurologic or mental disorder
B. Inconsistent decline in cognition, with no evidence of any other neurologic or mental disorder
C. Evidence of a cerebrovascular accident (CVA) and ataxia and poor speech
D. Visual field cuts and increased irritability

24. The nurse is gathering a history on a male 17-year-old patient accompanied by his parents. The patient's parents report concern for the patient's sudden onset of inattention, distractibility, fidgetiness in the classroom, and difficulty completing homework. With some symptoms consistent with attention deficit hyperactivity disorder (ADHD), the nurse understands that further screening is required if:

A. There were no noticeable concerns or symptoms in early childhood
B. The patient is male
C. The patient is a teenager
D. There is a family history of depression

(See answers next page.)

22. C) Amnesia
According to the *DSM-5,* the diagnosis for a neurocognitive disorder includes a TBI with one or more of the following: loss of consciousness, post-traumatic amnesia, disorientation and confusion, and neurological signs. Although anxiety, poor concentration, and headaches may exist with a TBI, these particular symptoms do not meet the criteria for a mild neurocognitive disorder.

23. A) Progressive decline in cognition, with no evidence of any other neurologic or mental disorder
According to the *DSM-5,* the diagnosis for Alzheimer disease must include clear evidence of a decline in memory or learning, a progressive and gradual decline in cognition, and no evidence of mixed etiology. Evidence of a CVA is an example of mixed etiology. Accompanying symptoms of a CVA are ataxia, poor speech, and visual field cuts. While irritability may be present with Alzheimer disease, it is not a marker for diagnostic criteria.

24. A) There were no noticeable concerns or symptoms in early childhood
According to the *DSM-5,* patients should show symptoms of ADHD before age 12 years. Given the patient's age, with no concerns prior to his current age, ADHD is not a probable diagnosis. Additional factors, including that the patient is male and a teenager, or if he has a family history of depression, would not be the most important predictors of a diagnosis of ADHD.

25. During assessment, a child is noticed to be messy and defiant. The psychiatric–mental health nurse's assessment of the patient's psychosexual stage according to Freud is:

A. Oral

B. Anal

C. Phallic

D. Latency

26. The common cognitive distortion that emphasizes the negative view and invalidates the positive view is known as:

A. All-or-nothing thinking

B. Labeling

C. Disqualifying the positive

D. Mind reading

27. A 7-year-old child shows a sense of being less than others. The child finds it difficult to learn and work. The psychological crisis exhibited is:

A. Trust versus mistrust

B. Autonomy versus shame and doubt

C. Industry versus inferiority

D. Intimacy versus isolation

28. The family member of a patient with schizophrenia reports that the patient has started to show signs of depression and has become apathetic and unmotivated. The nurse will assess how the patient's medication is affecting the system called:

A. Mesolimbic

B. Mesocortical

C. Nigrostriatal

D. Tuberoinfundibular

(See answers next page.)

25. B) Anal

The problematic traits seen in the anal stage of Freud's psychosexual stages are messiness, defiance, and rage. Traits in the oral stage include excessive dependency, envy, and jealousy. Phallic stage characteristics include sexual identity issues. The latency stage includes traits of excessive inner control.

26. C) Disqualifying the positive

Disqualifying the positive is the distortion that focuses on maintaining the negative view and disqualifying the positive view by marking it as irrelevant or inaccurate. "All-or-nothing" distortion makes the mind think in a black-and-white manner by reducing all complex outcomes. Labeling is a form of generalization and results in an overly harsh label for self or others. Mind reading is a type of distortion for jumping into negative interpretations.

27. C) Industry versus inferiority

Ages 6 to 12 years are characterized by developing social and physical skills and the ability to work efficiently. The child who is unable to develop these skills finds it difficult to learn and work and forms an inferiority complex, exhibiting the industry versus inferiority crisis. Trust versus mistrust is a psychological crisis that occurs in the age-group of 0 to 1½ years. Autonomy versus shame is characterized in the age-group of 18 months to 3 years. Intimacy versus isolation is characterized in the age-group of 20 to 35 years.

28. A) Mesolimbic

The mesolimbic pathway connects the ventral tegmental area to the nucleus accumbens and is associated with reward, motivation, and emotion. Mesocortical pathways are linked to cognitive function, executive function, and negative symptoms of schizophrenia. Nigrostriatal pathways are responsible for purposeful movement. The tuberoinfundibular pathway is responsible for the regulation of prolactin.

29. The 6-year-old patient's chief complaint is inattention. Attention deficit hyperactivity disorder. is suspected. The factors the nurse needs to consider when assessing for attention deficit disorder include absence of oppositional or defiant behavior, defiance, factors that may be related to medication, general medical condition, symptoms of hyperactivity/impulsivity, and the:

A. Length of time the symptom is reported, impact on function in more than one setting, and age of onset
B. Presence of episodic irritability, aggression, and grandiosity in the patient
C. Fact that the patient cannot soothe when angry, rages for hours, and is internally distracted
D. Patient's chronic irritable mood, with frequent explosive outbursts in more than one setting

30. An adult patient with no medical history of seizures reports being unable to sit still and concentrate on a given task. The patient also informs the nurse about frequent mood fluctuations. The nurse observes the patient talking very quickly and fidgeting constantly. The nurse suspects that the patient has symptoms that are related to which type of disorder?

A. Attention deficit hyperactivity
B. Personality
C. Mood
D. Cognitive

31. The dopamine and serotonin levels of the patient are lower than normal. The nurse should assess the patient for:

A. Mania
B. Depression
C. Anxiety
D. Narcolepsy

(See answers next page.)

29. A) Length of time the symptom is reported, impact on function in more than one setting, and age of onset

The chief complaint of inattention may be present in multiple diagnoses, such as oppositional defiant disorder, bipolar disorder, mood disorders, and disruptive mood dysregulation disorder (DMDD). It is often a challenge to differentiate among these disorders. The determining factors would include the age of onset, the length of time symptoms are present, and the impact on function in more than one setting. In order for a patient to be diagnosed with attention deficit hyperactivity disorder. The age of onset must be younger than age 12 years, with symptoms interfering with function in two or more settings. The presence of episodic irritability, aggression, and grandiosity suggests bipolar disorder. Inability to soothe when angry and raging for hours also suggests bipolar disorder. Chronic irritable mood with frequent explosive outbursts in more than one setting is indicative of DMDD. Patients with attention deficit disorder present with a more stable mood, are externally distracted, and are able to be soothed. Explosive outbursts are infrequent for both bipolar disorder and DMDD. Considering the differential diagnosis carefully is imperative because bipolar disorder may be worsened with the use of stimulants and carries a significant mortality risk.

30. A) Attention deficit hyperactivity

The patient is experiencing attention deficit hyperactivity disorder. The disorder is characterized by difficulty concentrating on particular tasks, impulsive behavior, mood fluctuations, and constant fidgeting. Personality disorders are marked by episodic changes in the behavior of an individual, with aggression as a diagnostic symptom. Mood disorders are a group of disorders that affect the mood of an individual, ranging from mania to depression. Cognitive disorders are characterized by changes in the thinking ability of an individual.

31. B) Depression

Levels of dopamine and serotonin remain low in cases of depression. In a patient with mania, levels of gamma-aminobutyric acid (GABA) decrease, while dopamine increases. Anxiety is characterized by increased levels of norepinephrine and low levels of GABA. Hypocretin levels remain increased in the case of narcolepsy.

32. A patient reports nausea and vomiting, tremors, dry mouth, sweating, and increased thirst, with onset 7 hours ago. The screening tool the nurse uses is the:

A. CAGE questionnaire
B. Patient Health Questionnaire
C. Insomnia Severity Index tool
D. Generalized Anxiety Disorders tool

33. An older adult patient visits the clinic with their spouse, who reports that the patient feels lonely and sad most of the time and does not eat well. Upon further assessment, it is revealed that the couple's daughter passed away 3 months ago. The best screening tool the nurse can use to further assess the symptoms is the:

A. Geriatric Depression Scale
B. Beck Depression Inventory
C. Strengths and Difficulties Questionnaire
D. Hospital Anxiety and Depression Scale

(See answers next page.)

32. A) CAGE questionnaire

The patient's symptoms and their duration lead the nurse to suspect alcohol withdrawal. The CAGE questionnaire is a tool used to screen for suspected alcohol misuse. It is administered by healthcare professionals. Item responses are scored 0 or 1, with the higher score being indicative of alcohol misuse. A total score of 2 or greater is considered clinically significant. If the screen is positive, the patient can be screened further with quantity and frequency questions. The Patient Health Questionnaire is a self-administered instrument for common mental health disorders. The Insomnia Severity Index tool is used for assessing the nature, severity, and impact of insomnia, and the Generalized Anxiety Disorders tool is used to assess anxiety disorders.

33. A) Geriatric Depression Scale

The Geriatric Depression Scale (GDS) is used for older adult patients. The GDS Long Form is a 30-item questionnaire to which participants are asked to respond by answering yes or no to questions about how they felt over the past week. A Short Form GDS consisting of 15 questions was developed in 1986. Questions from the Long Form GDS that had the highest correlation with depressive symptoms in validation studies were selected for the short version. Scores of 0 to 4 are considered normal, depending on age, education, and complaints; scores of 5 to 8 indicate mild depression; scores of 9 to 11 indicate moderate depression; and scores of 12 to 15 indicate severe depression. The Beck Depression Inventory is commonly used to assess patients for depression but would not be the most appropriate tool for older adults. The Strengths and Difficulties Questionaire is a self-evaluation tool for children with conduct and/or emotional problems. The Hospital Anxiety and Depression Scale is used to assess depression related to inpatient care.

2

Planning

1. The assertive community treatment team is meeting to compose a treatment plan for a new patient with bipolar disorder. To address the most common issue associated with long-term treatment, the primary focus of the treatment plan should be on:

   A. Increasing socialization
   B. Treatment compliance
   C. Obtaining employment
   D. Being accountable

2. The interdisciplinary team is conducting discharge planning for a patient newly diagnosed with bipolar disorder. In relation to the patient's diagnosis, which of the following requires investigation by the team?

   A. The patient lives in a small apartment with their intimate partner
   B. The patient has not discussed their diagnosis with their friends
   C. The patient works 12-hour night shifts at their job
   D. The patient would like to get pregnant sometime in the future

3. The spouse of a patient with borderline personality disorder (BPD) calls the clinic to report that the patient's behavior has not improved. Despite couples counseling, the patient is extremely moody and continues to blame the spouse for all of the issues in their marriage. The interdisciplinary team meets to review the patient treatment plan. Which of the following should the nurse recommend as the best therapy option for the patient at this time?

   A. Exposure therapy
   B. Dialectical behavioral therapy (DBT)
   C. Electroconvulsive therapy (ECT)
   D. Eye movement desensitization and reprocessing (EMDR)

(See answers next page.)

1. B) Treatment compliance

The most common issue seen with the treatment of patients with bipolar disorder is noncompliance. The team should primarily focus on measures that increase compliance, such as patient education, routine follow-ups, and establishing support systems. While socialization, employment, and accountability are all factors that are often impaired by bipolar disorder, consistent treatment of the underlying condition will address these aspects as well. Individually addressing socialization, employment, or accountability would not provide comprehensive care.

2. C) The patient works 12-hour night shifts at their job

To promote successful long-term treatment of bipolar disorder, the patient should implement lifestyle changes that contribute to a stable mood and minimize the risk for triggers. Working atypical hours, such as night shifts, results in the patient having an atypical schedule and will challenge the patient's ability to get the recommended amount of sleep. Working extended shifts, as in more than 8 hours, is known to be more stressful both physically and mentally. If possible, the patient should change to a job that facilitates a typical daytime schedule for stability. Living in a small apartment is acceptable as long as the accommodations are safe and meet the patient's needs. The acute focus is on the patient accepting their new diagnosis; the patient not being ready to discuss the diagnosis with friends is not concerning at this time. Many mental health medications are contraindicated during pregnancy; however, the patient does not want to get pregnant at the present time. The patient's medications and other treatment-related factors can be reviewed and altered when the patient reaches the point of being ready to try to conceive.

3. B) Dialectical behavioral therapy (DBT)

DBT has been shown to be particularly effective for patients with BPD, as it addresses behavior patterns as well as past experiences that have contributed to the condition. Exposure therapy would be useful for a patient with a severe phobia. ECT is a procedure that involves giving electrical stimulations to the brain and is used for severe, refractory cases of depression and bipolar disorder. EMDR is indicated for patients with a history of trauma. EMDR could address any trauma in the patient's past but does not help with behavioral modification, which is why it is not the recommended therapy option for this patient.

4. The nurse is providing discharge instructions to a patient who was admitted to an inpatient rehabilitation program for polysubstance use, including tobacco dependence, marijuana abuse, and MDMA/ecstasy use. The patient is being discharged home on sertraline (Zoloft). When educating the patient regarding the new medication, which of the following statements should the nurse include?

   A. "Using ecstasy with your medication can lead to a serious adverse reaction."
   B. "Cigarette smoking increases the risk for medication side effects."
   C. "Medical marijuana does not alter the effectiveness of the medication."
   D. "The medication will prevent you from being able to get high if you use drugs."

5. The nurse is working with a patient with post-traumatic stress disorder (PTSD) secondary to intimate partner violence. The patient is planning to leave their domestic partner. Which intervention recommended by the nurse can make the greatest difference between life and death for a patient who is experiencing intimate partner violence?

   A. Writing a list of safe houses and shelters along with contact information for these places
   B. Ensuring they have a least a month's worth of pay in savings before leaving the home
   C. Telling the abuser how much they care about them frequently to prevent episodes of abuse
   D. Keeping the children close by at all times to deflect episodes of physical abuse

6. The case management nurse for the psychiatric facility is arranging outpatient services for a patient with post-traumatic stress disorder (PTSD) secondary to experiences they had while in the military. Which service would the nurse select as the best option for this patient?

   A. Group therapy sessions that are specifically for veterans
   B. A general PTSD support group that meets via social media
   C. One-on-one support sessions with contemporary techniques
   D. Recorded videos that describe how to identify triggers

(See answers next page.)

4. A) "Using ecstasy with your medication can lead to a serious adverse reaction."

When combined with a selective serotonin reuptake inhibitor (SSRI) such as sertraline and MDMA/ecstasy can precipitate serotonin syndrome, which is a rare but serious medical emergency that results from high levels of serotonin in the body. Cigarette smoking is always discouraged, but it does not influence medication side effects. Marijuana, even if medicinal, can also cause serotonin syndrome. While the experience may be different, the medication does not prevent the patient from being able to get high if they use illicit substances.

5. A) Writing a list of safe houses and shelters along with contact information for these places

The risk of homicide by an intimate partner significantly rises when the patient leaves the home. Because of this, the patient should have a list of safe houses and shelters readily available to ensure they have a refuge when and if they decide to leave the home. While it would be ideal for the patient to have a significant amount of money saved before leaving the home, the patient should not remain in an unsafe environment because of money. Telling the abuser that they are cared about can improve or worsen the situation depending on the individual; there is no guarantee this will alter the behavior. Children should not witness abuse if at all possible and are often receivers of the abuse themselves.

6. A) Group therapy sessions that are specifically for veterans

Because of the unique and traumatic experiences of veterans, group activities such as support groups work best when the group members share similar backgrounds. This promotes comfort among the participants, which leads to sharing and understanding. A support group that provides general PTSD support services would include patients with various types of past traumas; a veterans-only group would be the preferred intervention. One-on-one sessions could be beneficial, but there is no guarantee the patient will feel comfortable discussing their experiences directly with the new provider. Also, there is nothing that indicates contemporary techniques are needed or have been requested by the patient. Recorded videos are helpful but would be used as an adjunct to support sessions, not a replacement. Videos do not engage the patient in the dialogue that is important in the healing process.

7. The nurse is arranging community-based services for a school-age patient. Which external factor would have the greatest impact on successful outcomes associated with these services?

   A. Housing type
   B. Current grade level
   C. Number of siblings
   D. Transportation

8. A patient with a history of opioid misuse has completed an inpatient treatment program. Based on the patient's history and current clinical status, the provider has placed an order to admit the patient to the hospital's intensive outpatient program (IOP). The patient asks how the IOP is different from going to regular counseling and support groups. Which of the following is the most appropriate response by the nurse?

   A. "They are almost identical. The only difference is that you can see your provider through IOP."
   B. "It is similar to the hospital's service except you are free during the day and sleep at the IOP."
   C. "You will receive all of the services you mentioned but on a much more frequent basis."
   D. "IOP primarily consists of medical services such as medication management."

9. A patient presents to the clinic with a new onset of severe depression. The patient is very anxious about the visit and asks if they can just get a prescription and leave. Which of the following would be the most appropriate response by the nurse?

   A. "You can complete these screening tools and immediately get a prescription."
   B. "You have the right to refuse evaluation by the provider and then receive medication."
   C. "You may need to have additional testing done to look for other conditions first."
   D. "You will not receive any prescriptions until you attend a couple of follow-up visits."

(See answers next page.)

7. D) Transportation

When planning outpatient services, it is important that the nurse ensure that the patient will be able to access the services. Treatment success in an outpatient community setting is dependent on the patient participating in services on a consistent basis. This patient must rely on family members, caregivers, and friends for transportation to the service location, which is why it is important to discuss transportation. The location of the patient's home could be a factor as it relates to transportation; however, the type of housing would not have a significant impact on the overall success. The treatment team who will be providing the community-based services will take grade level and family dynamics into consideration when planning care, but those are not external factors.

8. C) "You will receive all of the services you mentioned but on a much more frequent basis."

The primary difference between standard outpatient treatment and IOP treatment is the intensity of services. IOPs require attendance 3 to 5 times per week for several weeks. Depending on the individual IOP, patients may be able to see their provider through the program, but the services are vastly different from an inpatient program, which provides things such as continuous supervision. IOPs are usually held in the daytime hours; patients do not sleep at the IOP location. While some IOPs may integrate medical services such as medication management and laboratory testing, medical services are not the primary focus of the program.

9. C) "You may need to have additional testing done to look for other conditions first."

When planning care for a patient with a new onset of a mental health condition, a full psychiatric evaluation is required. Often, diagnostic testing is ordered to rule out underlying conditions such as thyroid issues. The screening tools administered to patients screen for symptoms of a specific mental health condition; they do not supply sufficient information to provide a formal diagnosis or determine the necessary treatment. Patients have the right to refuse aspects of care. The patient can refuse the evaluation; however, treatment cannot be prescribed until an evaluation is completed. If this were an involuntary admission, the patient would not be able to refuse the evaluation. Prescriptions are written at the time in which the provider feels sufficient information is present to correctly prescribe medications, which may or may not be at the first visit. There is no requirement that the patient has to complete a set number of follow-up visits before receiving a prescription.

10. The nurse is attending an interdisciplinary meeting for a new patient with a history of schizophrenia. Little information about the patient is available, and the patient is not able to logically communicate information at this time. Which of the following will the nurse investigate first, to assess for the most urgent issue that is prevalent in this patient population?

A. Living arrangements
B. Limited intellectual abilities
C. Body image disturbances
D. Inability to form a relationship

11. The nurse is working with a patient who has been hospitalized numerous times and is unable to care for themselves even when properly treated. The nurse consults the social worker and requests that they assist the patient in obtaining ongoing financial assistance and health insurance coverage from the:

A. Facility's administrative team
B. Social Security Administration (SSA)
C. Internal Revenue Service (IRS)
D. State Medicaid program

12. A patient who is 2 weeks postpartum arrives in the psychiatric emergency department. The patient has a history of postpartum depression, but the OB/GYN provider noted the patient's behavior to be atypical and referred the patient to the facility for evaluation. The patient has a flat affect and appears withdrawn but is cooperative. Which of the following should the nurse do to promote a therapeutic environment for the patient?

A. Tell the staff members not to discuss the newborn with the patient
B. Ensure that there is an available breast pump on the unit
C. Allow the spouse to bring the baby into the unit for visits
D. Ask the patient to use tampons instead of feminine hygiene pads

(See answers next page.)

10. A) Living arrangements

Homelessness is extremely prevalent among patients with schizophrenia because of a number of factors, including lack of adequate treatment and limited resources. The most pressing issue in planning for care of this patient is to identify the patient's current living situation because discharge planning will generally depend on where the patient will be residing. Limited intellectual abilities may be seen in patients with schizophrenia, but not all patients have these deficits. Body image disturbances can occur with any mental illness; however, that is not specific to this patient population and is not the most urgent issue. Patients with schizophrenia largely have the ability to form relationships. The challenge becomes maintaining relationships when mental health symptoms are poorly controlled or misunderstood by others.

11. B) Social Security Administration (SSA)

Patients who are disabled for medical and/or mental health reasons can apply for benefits from the SSA. Benefits available through the SSA include health insurance and a monthly monetary benefit that is paid to the patient. Some hospitals have programs that discount the cost of services based on the patient's income, but this is not insurance coverage, and it does not provide financial assistance. The IRS does not oversee federal disability programs or benefits. State Medicaid programs provide insurance coverage for certain patient populations; however, they do not provide financial assistance.

12. B) Ensure that there is an available breast pump on the unit

Planning for the needs of this patient includes recognizing any needs that are specific to a postpartum patient. If the patient is currently breastfeeding, the patient should be given the tools and space needed to pump breast milk. Even if the patient is prescribed medications during the hospital stay that are not recommended while breastfeeding, continuing to pump maintains breast milk production, which is important if the patient plans to resume breastfeeding upon discharge. Patients with postpartum depression and postpartum psychosis have varying views of their babies. If the patient brings up their baby and the conversation is appropriate, the staff can engage in a discussion involving the baby. Children are not allowed on acute psychiatric units because of safety reasons; this would also apply to a newborn. Identifying the needs of this patient involves recognizing associated medical needs as well. To prevent infection and ensure appropriate postpartum vaginal bleeding, feminine hygiene pads are to be used throughout the postpartum period; tampons should not be used during this time.

13. A patient who is preparing for discharge from the psychiatric hospital voices concerns about their job. The patient is an attorney and is professionally obligated to report the hospitalization to the licensing board. Which is the most appropriate response by the nurse?

A. "Your mental health condition will be an ongoing issue, so another career may be ideal."
B. "Required reporting is a form of discrimination and you should contact an attorney."
C. "If you feel you are mentally stable, you do not have to report it."
D. "The social worker can provide documentation to go with the report."

14. The nurse is planning care for a patient with autism spectrum disorder (ASD). The patient is scheduled to leave the facility for diagnostic testing and must be accompanied by a staff member. Which member of the care team should be assigned to the patient?

A. The nurse who was assigned to the patient yesterday
B. A mental health tech of the same cultural background
C. The charge nurse who is experienced with ASD
D. The unit's social worker who has a child with ASD

15. A male nurse is caring for a female patient in the psychiatric emergency department. The patient presented with depression and suicidal ideation. The patient interacts appropriately with her husband but does not respond to any of the questions asked by the nurse. There are no signs of abuse. The husband reports that in their culture, women are submissive and can interact with no men except for their husbands. What is the most appropriate action by the nurse?

A. Ensure patient safety, leave the room, and request that the patient be assigned a female nurse
B. Explain that due to the severity of symptoms, staffing changes are not possible
C. Report the husband's comments to the provider and social worker
D. Continue as the patient's nurse and obtain all information from the husband

(See answers next page.)

13. D) "The social worker can provide documentation to go with the report."

For public safety, there are professions that require self-disclosure of certain situations, including a psychiatric hospitalization. The patient should report the hospitalization, and social services can promote patient advocacy by providing documentation that can positively influence the report, such as patient compliance reports and the provider's prognosis projections. The goal of mental health treatment is to help the patient reach their optimal level of functioning, including returning to their career if desired. Professional reporting is used as a measure of public safety and is not a discrimatory activity. Mental stability as it pertains to the patient's professional obligations will be determined by the licensing board; at no time should the nurse recommend being noncompliant with reporting requirements.

14. A) The nurse who was assigned to the patient yesterday

Patients with ASD respond better in situations where there are familiar people and/or surroundings. The nurse who cared for the patient yesterday has established a relationship with the patient and would be the staff member the patient is most familiar with. Sharing the same cultural background may be comforting to the patient; however, the patient has already established a relationship with the previous nurse. While the charge nurse may have experience with the disorder, they are not the staff member with the most experience with this specific patient. The social worker who has a child with ASD could have difficulty separating care of the patient and their personal life.

15. A) Ensure patient safety, leave the room, and request that the patient be assigned a female nurse

The culturally competent nurse understands that there are varying beliefs among cultures. The belief that women are submissive and should act accordingly is a known principle in some cultures; a female nurse should be assigned to the patient if possible. Staffing changes can be made, even in the face of suicidal ideation, if it improves overall patient care. The patient is interacting appropriately with the spouse, and no evidence of abuse has been found, so there is no need to involve the provider or social worker. Ideally, information should be obtained directly from the patient and in the patient's own words. Obtaining information from the husband would be a secondary option if the patient did not communicate with the female nurse.

16. Upon discharge, a patient is prescribed cariprazine (Vraylar) for the treatment of refractory bipolar disorder. The patient reports they were prescribed this medication in the past but stopped taking it because of the cost. What is the first action the nurse should take?

    A. Advise the patient that this is the best treatment option and encourage them to ask their family members to assist with cost
    B. Contact the prescribing provider and ask that the patient be prescribed their previous medication regimen because of the cost
    C. Call the social worker and notify them of the patient's possible inability to obtain the prescribed medication
    D. Provide the patient with 30 days' worth of medication samples to allow time for them to find money for the medication

17. The nurse is working with the activities director to plan indoor activities for a substance use unit. What activity would the nurse identify as being the most appropriate for a patient admitted with methamphetamine use and severe skin picking who is experiencing withdrawal symptoms?

    A. Watching a movie on substance use
    B. Playing card games with the mental health tech
    C. Participating in a dance party in the cafeteria
    D. Reading a book on the patient's favorite topic

18. The nurse is preparing medications for a patient with extreme paranoia. In planning for administration of the medication, which action should the nurse take?

    A. Request a PRN ("as needed") order for forced medications
    B. Explain to the patient that the medication must be taken
    C. Point out other patients who are taking the same medication
    D. Allow the patient to open the pill packaging

(See answers next page.)

16. C) Call the social worker and notify them of the patient's possible inability to obtain the prescribed medication

The cost of the medication should be considered when a new medication is prescribed. If the patient cannot afford the prescribed medication, they will not be compliant with treatment. The social worker can work with the patient to obtain assistance with medication costs in a number of ways, including using assistance programs from the drug manufacturer and completing insurance prior authorizations if needed. If the patient is going to be discharged home on the medication, a solid plan for paying for the medication should be established; assistance from the family may be an option but is not guaranteed. The provider has prescribed the treatment option they feel is most appropriate, so the nurse should not recommend the previous medication regimen. The nurse would contact the provider if the treatment team is unable to secure assistance with medication cost. The patient should not be started on the medication until the team has ensured that the patient will be able to continue the treatment. If the medication is started using samples, but the patient cannot afford to continue the medication, it will lead to an abrupt stop of the medication, which comes with significant consequences.

17. B) Playing card games with the mental health tech

Patients with a history of skin picking or trichotillomania (hair pulling) have increased behaviors in settings where they are idle and/or bored. Playing cards with a mental health tech would occupy the patient's hands and reduce skin picking during the activity. Watching a movie and reading a book are sedentary activities that would create a setting where skin picking is likely. A dance party involves loud music, which may be overstimulating for a patient who is going through withdrawal symptoms.

18. D) Allow the patient to open the pill packaging

To facilitate cooperation by the patient, the nurse should allow the patient to participate in their care when it can be done safely. Allowing the patient to open the pill package and remove the pill can help ease the patient's paranoia because the patient can verify the medication they are being given. Forced medications should be a last resort, only after all other techniques have been unsuccessful. Telling the patient that the medication must be taken insinuates that the patient does not have a choice and can worsen the paranoia. Pointing out other patients breaches their confidentiality and is not known to eliminate paranoia in an unfamiliar situation.

19. A patient with a history of schizophrenia is experiencing psychosis and is very untrusting of the staff and other patients. What staff behavior will the nurse recommend to promote a therapeutic environment for the patient?

A. Ensure there is continuous activity to distract the patient
B. Avoid whispering and laughing at the nurses' station
C. Keep the patient in seclusion except for meal times
D. Frequently change the staff member assigned to the patient

20. A patient with a history of sexual abuse presents to the psychiatric emergency department with a panic attack. To provide the safest environment possible, the nurse should allow the patient to:

A. Select the nurse they would like to care for them
B. Sit in another patient's room to keep from being alone
C. Decide when they will be discharged home
D. Be admitted to the hospital under their sibling's name

21. During a home visit, the caregiver of a patient with late Alzheimer disease expresses safety concerns. They report that the patient has been getting up at night, and they have found the patient sitting outside on two occasions. What intervention should the nurse recommend to promote a safe environment?

A. Change the handle on the patient's bedroom door to enable the caregiver to lock the patient in
B. Relocate the locks on the doors leading outside to the top of the door
C. Administer the patient's prescribed sleeping pill at a later time of night
D. Have family members take turns staying up at night to check on the patient

(See answers next page.)

19. B) Avoid whispering and laughing at the nurses' station

Impaired perception of reality, distrust, and paranoia commonly occur with psychosis. The nurse should advise staff members to refrain from whispering or laughing at the nurses' station because the patient may think the staff members are talking about them. Continuous activity is not recommended because it can overstimulate the patient, worsening the psychosis. Seclusion is reserved for harmful behavior that cannot be addressed with any other intervention. Frequently changing the assigned staff member limits the amount of time spent with the patient, which prevents the staff member from establishing a trusting relationship.

20. A) Select the nurse they would like to care for them

When caring for a patient with a history of trauma or abuse, the nurse should implement measures that help eliminate triggers that could worsen the patient's current mental health symptoms. Allowing the patient to select their nurse provides the patient with the opportunity to identify the person whom they are most comfortable with, thus reducing the potential for a triggering situation. Allowing the patient to sit in another patient's room would breach confidentiality and should not be permitted. The patient will be discharged home when medically appropriate. Even if requested by the patient, discharge does not occur until the patient is deemed safe to leave the facility. If the patient does not want anyone to know they are in the facility, the hospital has processes that prevent the patient's admission from being discovered, such as not listing the patient's name in the public hospital census. Registering the patient under another person's name would be considered fraudulent activity.

21. B) Relocate the locks on the doors leading outside to the top of the door

Relocating the locks on doors leading to the outside to a high position removes the lock from the patient's direct line of sight. Also, as Alzheimer disease progresses, patients tend to forget to look up. A highly placed lock may also be out of the patient's reach. Locking the patient in their room is unsafe and highly inappropriate because the patient is not able to access things that are needed to meet their basic needs, such as toileting, food, and water. The patient is also unable to contact others if assistance is needed. The patient's behavior is due to their condition; therefore, it would not be corrected by changing the timing of their night medication. Having family members take turns staying up at night places a significant burden on the family and would not be sustainable. The goal would be to implement measures that directly impact the patient's behavior.

22. The nurse is preparing decorations for the month of December and would like to hang a banner above the door. Which of the following would the nurse select as the most appropriate signage for the upcoming holiday?
    A. Merry Christmas
    B. Happy holidays
    C. Celebrate Hanukkah
    D. Happy Kwanzaa

23. The nurse is coordinating a day program for patients with various mental health conditions. The patients are rewarded with a movie after certain benchmarks are reached. Which approach should the nurse take when planning the movie sessions?
    A. The nurse should always pick the movie based on the newest release
    B. The patients should rotate picking a movie from the facility's library
    C. The patients should nominate the person to pick the movie each day
    D. The patient should take turns bringing in a movie from home

24. Shampoo and hair conditioner are provided to all patients admitted to the inpatient psychiatric facility. A patient approaches the nurse and states that they have asked their family member to bring their hair products to the facility. The patient uses hair products appropriate for their hair type according to ethnicity. Which of the following is the most appropriate action by the nurse?
    A. Call the family member and cancel the patient's request for hair products
    B. Allow the patient to keep the hair products in their room so other patients do not see them
    C. Make the hair products available for use of all patients on the unit
    D. Store the hair products at the nurses' station and allow use with supervision

25. A patient with severe anxiety and depression is enrolled in an outpatient program. The patient recently started taking college courses and reports that their anxiety is worse when they are in class. When updating the patient's treatment plan, the nurse understands that the patient may be eligible for which of the following treatment adjuncts?
    A. Parking in the front of building
    B. Stimulant medications
    C. Grade curve based on diagnosis
    D. Emotional support animal

(See answers next page.)

22. B) Happy holidays
Unit activities, including hanging decorations, should always be as inclusive as possible. The term "happy holidays" encompasses all of the various holidays that occur during this time of year and would be the most appropriate. While Christmas is the most widely celebrated December holiday in the United States, it is a religious holiday, and the nurse should not assume that all patients celebrate it. Because Hanukkah and Kwanzaa are religious and/or cultural holidays, they would not be the best choice for decorations because not all patients celebrate these holidays.

23. B) The patients should rotate picking a movie from the facility's library
The nurse should plan for the patients to take turns picking a movie so that all patients feel involved and are treated equally. Having the nurse pick each movie does not ensure the movie will be of interest to the patients; there is no reason why the newest release should be selected. Allowing the patients to choose the person who will select the movie may isolate other patients. The nurse must ensure that the movie content is appropriate, so movies should routinely be selected from the approved library rather than brought from patients' homes.

24. D) Store the hair products at the nurses' station and allow use with supervision
When specific cultural needs present themselves, the nurse should make every effort to meet those needs if it is safe to do so. Requesting specific hair products according to ethnicity, not for cosmetic purposes, is a reasonable request. The products should be held at the nurses' station and used only at appropriate times with staff supervision. Because the request can be safely accommodated, the nurse should not call the family member to cancel. For patient safety, the products should be stored at the nurses' station with the other hygiene products. The products being used are allowed for cultural reasons so there is no reason to offer the products to other patients.

25. D) Emotional support animal
An emotional support animal is an option for this patient based on their diagnosis if the presence of the animal lessens the mental health symptoms. Accommodations such as parking in front of the building are usually reserved for physical disabilities that make it difficult to walk longer distances. Stimulant medications are used to treat attention deficit hyperactivity disorder and can worsen anxiety. Classroom interventions are possible based on the patient's individual needs; however, there are no accommodations that would adjust the patient's grade based on their diagnosis alone.

26. The nurse is caring for a patient who presented to the psychiatric emergency department for suicidal ideation. The patient's current appearance is more traditionally feminine than their driver's license photograph. The patient confirms that the identifying information on the license is correct. How should the nurse initially address the situation?

A. Ask the patient if they are really a boy or a girl
B. Request an order for male hormone testing
C. Question the patient about their sexual orientation
D. Clarify the patient's preferred pronouns

27. The nurse recognizes the importance of appropriate mental health services for patients in the LGBTQ+ community, understanding that different mental health conditions are more prevalent in certain patient populations. Which of the following is the the most important factor to initally assess when planning care specifically for transgender patients?

A. Intimate relationships
B. Suicidal thoughts
C. Impulse control
D. Social interactions

28. The nurse is admitting a new patient to the psychiatric facility when the patient's adult child arrives, demanding that their parent be released from the facility. The nurse explains that the patient was found in their home, which was extremely dirty and did not have running water. No food was found in the home. The patient stated to the responders that the findings were normal for them and that they did not see what the problem was. The adult child states that the patient has not tried to harm themself or anyone else and again demands that the nurse discharge the patient. How should the nurse proceed?

A. Move forward with the admission of the patient
B. Request the patient be discharged to the care of the adult child
C. Transfer the patient to a medical facility for evaluation
D. Terminate the admission because of the absence of threats of harm

(See answers next page.)

26. D) Clarify the patient's preferred pronouns

Gender identity is an important factor for the nurse to assess because it is critical to the patient's personal awareness. The patient's identifying information has been confirmed, so the next step would be for the nurse to ask for the patient's preferred pronouns to ensure they are addressed in an appropriate and respectful manner. If there is a question about the patient's sex or genitalia as it relates to treatment, the patient should be asked about their biological sex or sex assigned at birth. The terms "boy" and "girl" should not be used. Regardless of gender, hormone testing is not indicated in this situation. Gender identity and sexual orientation are two different elements and should be addressed separately. The nurse can ask about sexual orientation at a later time if the information is pertinent to care.

27. B) Suicidal thoughts

The prevelance of suicidal ideation and suicide attempts is high in the transgender population. While other factors are important, assessing for suicidal thoughts would be the priority. Intimate partner violence can be seen in all populations and is not specific to transgender patients. Assessing for impulse control would be important for patients with mental health conditions such as mood disorders but would not be specific to the transgender population. Social interactions should be included with all mental health assessments, not just with those of transgender patients.

28. A) Move forward with the admission of the patient

An involuntary admission can be ordered if the patient is a threat to themselves, a threat to someone else, or gravely disabled, meaning that they cannot meet their basic needs. The patient meets the criteria for an involuntary admission, and the nurse should move forward with the admission as ordered. Because the patient meets criteria for an involuntary admission, the patient can be discharged only when it is ordered by a provider; it would not be appropriate for the nurse to request discharge at this time. A medical facility would not be the appropriate place to evaluate the psychiatric issue the patient is presenting with. While there are no known threats of harm, the patient is gravely disabled, so terminating the admission would be an inappropriate action.

29. The facility's activity coordinator has planned a group activity where each patient on the pediatric unit will make a Mother's Day card in preparation for the upcoming holiday. How should the nurse proceed with the planned activity?

A. Suggest the patients learn how to make various origami shapes with paper
B. Arrange the patients into small groups so that they can share supplies
C. Provide the name of each child's mother to personalize the cards
D. Recommend teaching the patients how to knit gifts for their mothers

30. A school-age patient is preparing to transition home after a 6-month inpatient stay. The interdisciplinary team has been working with the patient's parent to ensure a smooth transition. Which of the following statements by the parent would indicate that further planning is needed?

A. "I have arranged to have all of my child's friends here when they arrive home."
B. "I have asked my child what type of snacks they would like at home."
C. "I have removed items in the home that previously triggered my child."
D. "I have spoken to the guidance counselor about the transition back to school."

31. A patient has been hospitalized for 7 days because of violent public outbursts. The social work team has arranged for discharge in the morning to a home for veterans. The patient has a history of post-traumatic stress disorder and alcohol use disorder. The patient's mental status and behavior have both improved overall, but the patient still has mild outbursts that are easily triggered. The nurse administered the first dose of disulfiram (Antabuse) today. How should the nurse proceed with the current discharge plan?

A. Explain to the patient the steps they will experience during discharge in the morning
B. Advise the social work team that the patient cannot be discharged on disulfiram
C. Call the home for veterans and let them know the patient is still having outbursts
D. Arrange a meeting with the interdisciplinary team to discuss the pending discharge

(See answers next page.)

29. A) Suggest the patients learn how to make various origami shapes with paper

When planning activities, the treatment team must consider various patient circumstances. There is no guarantee that all of the patients have a mother or that all of the patients have a positive relationship with their mothers. An activity that would be appropriate for all of the patients would be an activity not specific to Mother's Day, such as origami. Sharing supplies, disclosing the names of the patients' mothers, and knitting a Mother's Day gift would not be indicated because the planned activity involving Mother's Day needs to be changed to a more general activity. Also, knitting involves sharp objects, which would create a safety issue on the unit.

30. A) "I have arranged to have all of my child's friends here when they arrive home."

Transitioning home after any admission, particularly a longer inpatient stay, can be stressful and anxiety producing. Having multiple people present when the patient initially returns home can be overwhelming for the patient. The parent should arrange for only close family and/or the people the patient has requested to be present upon arrival. Providing preferred snacks promotes the patient being more comfortable at home. Removing previous triggers helps prevent negative emotional responses. The guidance counselor should be involved to ensure an appropriate transition back into the classwork.

31. D) Arrange a meeting with the interdisciplinary team to discuss the pending discharge

Based on their current status, the patient is not ready for discharge to a nonmedical facility, and the nurse should arrange a meeting with the interdisciplinary team to discuss the concerns about the pending discharge. The patient is easily triggered, which could create a significant issue in a veterans' home where the residents are sensitive to such behavior. Also, the patient has only received one dose of disulfiram (Antabuse), so more time is needed to assess whether the patient will tolerate the medication. The nurse should not discuss the anticipated steps of discharge with the patient at this time; the discussion should take place after the nurse meets with the team to discuss the plan. Patients can be safely discharged home on disulfiram as long as they are educated on the medication and are tolerating the medication well. A full report, including information on the outbursts, should be given to the veterans' home staff once the discharge date is confirmed with the treatment team.

32. A pediatric Spanish-speaking patient comes into the office for an initial visit with parents who speak only Spanish. The nurse practices cultural competence by:

A. Using another family member as an interpreter
B. Using language services to provide an interpreter
C. Moving forward with the patient without an interpreter
D. Using a few known Spanish words to enhance the patient's understanding

(See answers next page.)

32. B) Using language services to provide an interpreter
Using an authorized interpreter demonstrates cultural competence, with an awareness of the need to enhance the patient's (and parents') understanding and communication with the provider to provide appropriate care. Family members should not be used as interpreters because of patient confidentiality and the need to ensure that accurate information is being relayed to and from the patient. The nurse is not practicing cultural competence if continuing without an interpreter or attempting to communicate with the patient in a language in which they are not fluent.

3

Implementation

1. The nurse is performing an assessment on an 8-year-old patient who is prescribed clonidine (Catapres) for a mental health condition. Which of the following should the nurse use to measure the desired outcome?

   A. Blood pressure and pulse
   B. Patient Health Questionnaire–9 (PHQ-9)
   C. Mood Disorder Questionnaire (MDQ)
   D. ADHD Rating Scale–5

2. A newly admitted patient with a diagnosis of bulimia nervosa arrives in the cafeteria for lunch. To ensure a safe environment, the nurse should:

   A. Request a liquid diet for all meals
   B. Seat the patient at a table alone
   C. Assign a tech to the patient after the meal is over
   D. Schedule future meals in the patient's room

3. A patient with a history of bipolar I is admitted to the psychiatric hospital because of a manic episode. The patient is extremely hyperactive and has difficulty sitting still. The nurse notices that the patient has eaten very little for breakfast and lunch. Which of the following would be an appropriate action by the nurse to improve the patient's dietary intake?

   A. Do not allow the patient to leave the cafeteria until they have consumed at least 50% of their meal
   B. Administer an as-needed sedative immediately prior to meals to help calm the patient
   C. Request an order from the provider for an appetite stimulant before meals
   D. Submit a dietary request for the patient to have chicken nuggets and fries for dinner

(See answers next page.)

1. D) ADHD Rating Scale–5

Clonidine is commonly prescribed to pediatric patients for the treatment of attention deficit hyperactivity disorder (ADHD). The ADHD Rating Scale–5 can be used to quickly determine the severity of ADHD symptoms in children and adolescents. Clonidine is not used to treat depression or mood disorders in children; therefore, the PHQ-9 tool, which assesses symptoms of depression, and the MDQ, which screens for mood disorders, would not be useful. While measuring blood pressure and pulse would be part of the general patient assessment, the medication was not prescribed for blood pressure management, so blood pressure and pulse readings would not evaluate the intended outcomes. In addition, clonidine can only be prescribed to children age 12 years and older for the treatment of hypertension.

2. C) Assign a tech to the patient after the meal is over

The hallmark activities associated with bulimia nervosa are episodes of binge eating followed by inappropriate behaviors to avoid gaining weight—most commonly, vomiting after meals. Assigning a mental health tech to the patient after the meal is over helps deter the unhealthy activity of post-meal vomiting. There is no medical reason for the patient to have a liquid diet because the behaviors are not related to the consistency of food. Having the patient sit alone unnecessarily isolates the patient and does not provide any benefit to their condition. Allowing the patient to eat meals in their room increases the opportunity for bulimic behaviors and should be avoided.

3. D) Submit a dietary request for the patient to have chicken nuggets and fries for dinner

During a manic episode, patients find it difficult to complete tasks that require sitting for any length of time, such as eating meals. Chicken nuggets and fries are finger foods that can be eaten on the go and do not require the patient to sit still to consume them. The inability to sit still for meals is due to the current mental state; it is not a deliberate choice. Requiring the patient to stay in the cafeteria would only be an option if the patient was able to make the decision to sit and finish the meal. Administering a sedative would not be appropriate in this situation because the patient is not demonstratting behaviors that present a safety concern. Also, administering a sedative prior to the patient eating creates a risk for choking and aspiration. An appetite stimulant is not needed; the loss of appetite is due to the manic episode and will naturally improve as the mania subsides.

4. A patient with schizophrenia begins screaming at the nurse, demanding that the nurse tell the person sitting next to them to stop talking. There is no one sitting next to the patient, and no one is talking to the patient. Which of the following is the correct response by the nurse?

A. "I need more information about the conversation. Come sit by me so that I can listen to what they are saying."

B. "Sit down and try to stay calm. I'm calling security to remove that person right now."

C. "I understand that you hear someone talking; I do not see anyone around you at this time."

D. "I have already explained that the voices you are hearing are not real. No one is talking to you."

5. A patient with borderline personality disorder (BPD) asks the nurse to go outside for an extra smoke break. The nurse tells the patient they have already had all of their allowed smoke breaks for the day. The patient states, "The day shift nurse is much nicer than you are because they let me have an extra break to calm my nerves. They told me the night shift staff was lazy." What is the most appropriate action by the nurse?

A. Make a one-time exception now but do not allow any future exceptions

B. Discuss that the workload for the day shift and the night shift is the same

C. Advise the patient to return to their room and do not address the statements

D. Offer the patient a nicotine patch and review the smoke break rules

6. A patient with narcissistic personality disorder is participating in an outpatient treatment program. Today the patients are educated on therapeutic communication methods, then given a short quiz on what they have learned. Which action by the nurse could trigger a negative response from the patient?

A. Hanging all of the graded quizzes on the bulletin board

B. Meeting with the individual patient to discuss the answers

C. Generically reviewing the quiz with the group as a whole

D. Giving all of the patients the opportunity to retake the quiz

(See answers next page.)

4. C) "I understand that you hear someone talking; I do not see anyone around you at this time."

When a patient is experiencing hallucinations of any type, the nurse should acknowledge what the patient is experiencing and gently attempt to reorient the patient by clearly stating the reality of the situation in a unprovoking way. The nurse should never reinforce hallucinations, so telling the patient to sit close so that the nurse can listen to the conversation would not be appropriate. Calling security to remove a fictitious person would also be reinforcing the hallucination. Denying what the patient is experiencing is not therapeutic and leads to negative outcomes such as defensiveness, paranoia, and impaired nurse–patient relations.

5. D) Offer the patient a nicotine patch and review the smoke break rules

When caring for a patient with BPD, it is important that the nurse is consistent, establishes boundaries, and sets clear expectations. The patient is displaying manipulative behavior by pitting staff members against each other, which is consistent with BPD. Offering the patient a nicotine patch addresses the patient's reported need for nicotine to calm their nerves while staying within the rules of the facility. Reviewing the smoke break rules with the patient resets expectations and boundaries. Making an exception, even once, endorses the inappropriate behavior by the patient and should not be allowed. Discussing the workload for each shift is discouraged because the nurse should not engage in a conversation about rumored information; replying would give attention to the inappropriate statement. Instead of purposely not addressing the patient's request, the nurse should address it using appropriate communication; communicating expectations and setting boundaries are therapeutic interventions that aim to change the patient's behavior.

6. A) Hanging all of the graded quizzes on the bulletin board

The hallmark behaviors associated with narcissistic personality disorder include grandiose ideas, arrogance, a sense of entitlement, and an extremely positive self-image. By hanging the graded quizzes for public review, the nurse allows others to see the patient's wrong answers. Also, if other patients made a higher score, seeing this could invoke a negative reaction by the patient because of their inflated self-image. Providing a one-on-one quiz review would be appropriate as it allows time to review the material with the patient without letting others know about the quiz grade. A generic overview to the group does not point out any one patient's flaws and would be an acceptable action. Allowing any patient to retake the quiz provides them with the opportunity to make a better quiz grade, which would increase self-confidence.

7. An older adult patient with severe depression presents to the facility because of worsening depression with suicidal ideation. The patient has been prescribed a number of oral antidepressants in the past with minimal results. The patient has a history of chronic kidney disease, diabetes, and cirrhosis of the liver. If not previously tried, which would the nurse identify as a safe treatment option for this patient?

   A. Olanzapine (Zyprexa) monthly injection
   B. Paroxetine (Paxil) oral tablets
   C. Mirtazapine (Remeron SolTab)
   D. Electroconvulsive therapy (ECT)

8. The nurse is performing a home visit to administer a monthly injection of paliperidone palmitate (Invega Sustenna) to a patient with schizoaffective disorder. The caregiver reports that the patient is doing well on the medication and would like to know if there are any changes they can make to facilitate safe long-term treatment with the medication. What recommendation should the nurse provide to help prevent medication-associated adverse reactions?

   A. Implement a strict calorie-restriction diet to prevent weight gain
   B. Limit fluid intake to prevent edema or swelling
   C. Avoid eating aged cheeses and processed meats
   D. Practice daily carbohydrate counting with each meal

9. A patient who is prescribed fluoxetine (Prozac) capsules states that they cannot swallow pills because they have a fear of choking. Which of the following would be an appropriate action by the nurse?

   A. Open the capsule and sprinkle the medication on ice cream
   B. Advise the patient that their fear is not rational
   C. Discuss the consequences of being noncompliant
   D. Contact the provider regarding alternative forms of the medication

(*See answers next page.*)

7. D) Electroconvulsive therapy (ECT)
ECT has been found to be especially helpful in refractory major depressive disorder, even in the older adult population, making this a safe option for the patient. Olazapine and mirtazapine have convenient administration methods; however, being older, having a history of diabetes, and having hepatic impairment all make these medication options undesirable. Of all of the selective serotonin reuptake inhibitors (SSRIs), paroxetine has the longest half-life, which is a concern when administering the medication to a patient with renal impairment.

8. D) Practice daily carbohydrate counting with each meal
Paliperidone palmitate (Invega Sustenna) can cause hyperglycemia, diabetes mellitus, and extremes of glucose impairment such as ketoacidosis. Practicing carbohydrate counting is a simple, noninvasive way to maintain glucose control and reduce the risk of developing medication-induced hyperglycemia. The weight gain associated with taking antipsychotics is not the result of an excess in caloric intake. A strict calorie-restriction diet would be a harmful intervention because it can result in poor nutrition. The adverse reactions associated with the medication are not associated with excessive fluid intake. If swelling or edema develops as a result of the medication, it should be reported to the treatment team, as this would be a concerning finding. Foods such as aged cheeses and processed meats are high in tyramine and are prohibited in patients who are taking monoamine oxidase inhibitors (MAOIs).

9. D) Contact the provider regarding alternative forms of the medication
Contacting the provider regarding other forms of the medication will allow the patient to move forward with the prescribed medication while addressing the patient's fear of swallowing; fluoxetine comes as a liquid solution. The capsule is a delayed-release medication, so the capsules should never be opened because this changes the delivery of the medication. A fear of choking while taking a pill is understandable. While the chance of choking on a single capsule is very small, the patient's concerns should be addressed. The patient is objecting to having to swallow a pill; they are not refusing the medication at this time. If the patient continues to be unable to take the medication after a suitable replacement is offered, the nurse can reassess the patient's level of compliance.

10. An older patient is having severe difficulty sleeping since transferring to a new psychiatric treatment facility. The patient does not have a history of insomnia or difficulty sleeping. The provider has ordered trazodone, 50-mg tablets, one to two tablets by mouth at bedtime as needed for insomnia. What is the most appropriate action by the nurse?

A. Administer trazodone 50 mg by mouth
B. Schedule the trazodone for bedtime each night
C. Administer trazodone 100 mg by mouth
D. Discontinue the ordered trazodone

11. The nurse receives an order to continue the home medications for a new patient who is admitted for bipolar mania. Which medication should the nurse hold until it is discussed with the provider?

A. Divalproex sodium (Depakote)
B. Quetiapine (Seroquel)
C. Alprazolam (Xanax)
D. Lisdexamfetamine (Vyvanse)

12. The nurse on a geriatric psychiatric unit is working with a patient with depression. The patient has been quiet but cooperative since their admission. The nurse announces that it is time for a group session and requests that everyone go into the therapy room, but the patient remains seated. What is the most appropriate initial action by the nurse?

A. Document the patient's noncompliant behavior
B. Yell the instructions in the patient's direction
C. Repeat the instructions while standing in front of the patient
D. Administer an as-needed antianxiety medication to the patient

(See answers next page.)

10. A) Administer trazodone 50 mg by mouth
With all medications, especially medications administered to older patients, the nurse should apply the "start low and go slow" principle, which means the nurse will start with the lowest dose and gradually increase the dose until the desired effect is reached. The nurse should administer 50 mg of trazodone initially; a second tablet can be administered if the initial dose is not sufficient. The medication was ordered on an as-needed basis, so it should not be routinely scheduled each night. Not having a history of insomnia is a reason to start at a low dose; it is not a reason to discontinue the medication. The current clinical picture does not indicate a need to discontinue the prescribed medication.

11. D) Lisdexamfetamine (Vyvanse)
Lisdexamfetamine (Vyvanse) is a stimulant medication that is used to treat attention deficit hyperactivity disorder (ADHD). Because the medication is a stimulant, it has the potential to trigger or worsen symptoms of mania. The nurse should clarify this medication with the provider prior to administration. Divalproex sodium can be used as a mood stabilizer for patients with bipolar disorder and can be administered to this patient. Quetiapine has several indications, including bipolar mania, bipolar depression, anxiety, and insomnia, making it an appropriate medication option. The use of a benzodiazepine, such as alprazolam, for the treatment of anxiety symptoms as needed is acceptable.

12. C) Repeat the instructions while standing in front of the patient
When working with older adult patients, the nurse should be mindful of special considerations associated with the population. It is very common for geriatric patients to be hard of hearing, so the nurse should first repeat the instructions while standing in front of the patient to allow the patient the opportunity to acknowledge that the nurse is making a request and to read the nurse's lips if needed. The nurse should not immediately assume the patient is being noncompliant. Yelling at the patient can be perceived as embarrassing, demeaning, or intimidating; the nurse should speak directly into the patient's ear as opposed to yelling if they are concerned the patient did not hear the instructions. The patient has not demonstrated any behavior that suggests that the patient is anxious, making an antianxiety medication unnecessary at this time.

13. The nurse is administering the first dose of vilazodone (Viibryd) to a patient with depression. The patient states that they do not want to take the medication because of side effects they experienced with prior antidepressant medications. Further discussion reveals that the patient previously experienced significant sexual side effects that they feel negatively impacted their marriage. Which of the following would be an appropriate initial response by the nurse?

A. "Some antidepressants are known to cause sexual side effects; however, this medication has a much lower risk of causing sexual side effects."
B. "Sexual side effects are unavoidable with antidepressants, but your mental health is more important than decreased sexual desire."
C. "Sexual side effects are possible with any antidepressant medication, but they always go away eventually."
D. "The sexual side effects that you previously experienced were likely due to the medications prescribed for your medical conditions."

14. The nurse is reviewing treatment options that may address a nursing diagnosis of noncompliance for a patient with schizophrenia. The patient has been admitted to the psychiatric facility several times over the past year and is not compliant with their prescribed medication regimen. The patient reports that they do not have stable housing, which makes it difficult for them to keep up with their medications. Which of the following oral medications would best address the issue with compliance?

A. Olanzapine (Zyprexa)
B. Haloperidol (Haldol)
C. Ziprasidone (Geodon)
D. Quetiapine (Seroquel)

15. The nurse is obtaining a daily weight on a patient who is admitted with anorexia nervosa. The patient is very apprehensive about being weighed and states that they do not want to know how much they weigh. Based on the patient's reaction to being weighed, what is the most appropriate action by the nurse?

A. Change the order from daily weights to obtaining patient weight every other day
B. Allow the patient to weigh themselves and report the weight to the nurse
C. Ask the patient to step on the scale with their back facing the screen of the scale
D. Offer to skip today's weight if the patient consumes 50% of the next meal

(See answers next page.)

13. A) "Some antidepressants are known to cause sexual side effects; however, this medication has a much lower risk of causing sexual side effects."

Sexual side effects are commonly seen with antidepressant medications such as selective serotonin reuptake inhibitors (SSRIs) and serotonin and norepinephrine reuptake inhibitors (SNRIs). Vilazodone (Viibryd) is a serotonin modulator that acts differently on the central nervous system, significantly reducing the risk for sexual side effects. Telling the patient their mental health is more important minimizes the concerns the patient has voiced. Sexual side effects can improve and may resolve over time, but this is not the case for all patients. Regardless of the medical medications the patient may be prescribed, the nurse understands that antidepressants are a common cause of sexual side effects and should not deflect the concern.

14. A) Olanzapine (Zyprexa)

Because of the patient's history of noncompliance, a medication with once-a-day dosing and a longer half-life would be the best option. Of the medications listed, olanzapine has the longest half-life at over 20 hours. If the patient continues to be noncompliant on oral olanzapine, the patient can be transitioned to the injectable form of the medication, which is given every 2 to 4 weeks. Haloperidol also has a long half-life but it is taken 2 to 3 times a day, which increases the risk for noncompliance. Also, first-generation antipsychotics, such as haloperidol, have more side effects than second-generation antipsychotics. Ziprasidone and quetiapine are second-generation antipsychotics; however, the half-life of the oral versions of these medications is less than the half-life of olanzapine.

15. C) Ask the patient to step on the scale with their back facing the screen of the scale

Consistent and accurate weight monitoring is a critical aspect of the treatment plan for a patient with anorexia nervosa. These patients are overly concerned with their weight, so being weighed can be an anxiety-inducing experience for the patient. To help ease the associated anxiety, the nurse should weigh the patient with their back to the screen of the scale so that the weight cannot be viewed by the patient. The nurse can share the weight with the patient if they would like to know the result. The nurse cannot independently change the current order to obtaining the patient's weight every other day; daily weights are the most accurate method of measurement for this patient. A daily weight needs to be obtained regardless of how much of a meal the patient consumes. Offering to skip the ordered intervention in exchange for 50% meal consumption would be inappropriate.

16. The mental health technician reports that a patient has become agitated and is anxious. The patient is walking back and forth across the unit. Which is the most appropriate initial action by the nurse?

A. Tell the patient to sit down immediately so they can discuss how they are feeling

B. Administer an antianxiety medication, then attempt to discuss the symptoms

C. Walk with the patient across the unit while asking about their feelings

D. Place the patient in seclusion until they are able to control their anxiety

17. Naltrexone (Vivitrol) is prescribed for a patient with a history of alcohol use disorder. The patient is tall and has a body mass index (BMI) of 16.1. The patient has no medication allergies, and the medical history is positive for asthma. What action should the nurse take?

A. Update the prescribing provider with the risks associated with administration to this patient

B. Administer the medication as prescribed and assess for side effects in 1 hour

C. Auscultate for wheezing and administer the medication if wheezing is not present

D. Hold administration of the medication until the patient requests it to be administered

18. The nurse has administered a dose of sodium oxybate (Xyrem) to a patient with narcolepsy. The patient has used this medication in the past with good results and denies any previous side effects. Which of the following would be the most appropriate action by the nurse?

A. Instruct the patient to notify the nurse if they do not fall into deep sleep within an hour

B. Offer the patient a dose of an antianxiety medication with the medication to facilitate sleep

C. Automatically administer a second dose of sodium oxybate (Xyrem) by mouth in 3 to 4 hours

D. Place naloxone (Narcan) at the bedside to reverse the medication in case of respiratory depression

(See answers next page.)

16. C) Walk with the patient across the unit while asking about their feelings

When treating anxiety, it is important to address what is causing the anxiety, so it is important that the nurse discuss the symptoms with the patient. Being fidgety and being unable to keep still are symptoms associated with anxiety, and forcing the patient to suddenly stop that behavior without any other intervention can worsen the anxiety; therefore, the most appropriate initial step by the nurse would be to walk with the patient while discussing their anxiety episode. Asking the patient to immediately sit down can worsen the anxiety symptoms. An antianxiety medication may be needed, but the initial interventions would use nonpharmacological methods. Seclusion is reserved as a last resort for harmful behavior or behavior that presents a safety issue.

17. A) Update the prescribing provider with the risks associated with administration to this patient

Naltrexone (Vivitrol) is administered as an intramuscular injection and can be prescribed for the treatment of alcohol use disorder. It is important that the medication is administered into the muscle. If the medication is accidentally administered subcutaneously, a significant injection site reaction can occur; therefore, administration is not recommended if the medication cannot be given via deep intramuscular route. The nurse should notify the prescribing provider that the patient's body habitus places the patient at high risk for accidental subcutaneous administration. If the medication is administered, the nurse should assess for side effects, including respiratory symptoms such as wheezing; however, this would not take place until after the nurse has updated the provider with their concerns and the provider decides to move forward with the injection. The medication would not be administered, regardless of the patient's request, until the provider authorizes the administration after discussing it with the nurse.

18. C) Automatically administer a second dose of sodium oxybate (Xyrem) by mouth in 3 to 4 hours

Sodium oxybate (Xyrem) is prescribed for treatment of narcolepsy. The medication is administered orally, with the first dose being administered around bedtime and the second dose administered 2.5 to 4 hours after the first dose. Deep sleep is expected after administration of the second dose. To prevent potential medication interactions and side effects, no additional medications should be administered at the same time as the sodium oxybate (Xyrem). Naloxone cannot reverse the effects of sodium oxybate (Xyrem).

19. A patient who is prescribed propanolol for performance anxiety asks the nurse for a dose of the medication prior to going to group therapy. Which of the following findings should the nurse report to the prescribing provider prior to administering the medication?

A. Blood pressure 120/78
B. History of asthma
C. Apical pulse of 105
D. Pravastatin allergy

20. A patient was prescribed zolpidem (Ambien) for insomnia due to trouble sleeping after the death of a close friend. The previous nurse documented that they found the patient in the kitchen eating while still asleep. What action should the nurse take in regard to the medication?

A. Cut the dose in half for the first 2 weeks, then increase to the full dose
B. Prevent access to the kitchen at night by using barriers and blocking doors
C. Stop the medication, then assess to see if the sleep-eating behavior continues
D. Schedule the dose of the medication around dinnertime so that others are around while the patient is eating

21. A patient began to remove their clothes while in the common area of the unit. When asked to put their clothes back on, the patient physically attacked the staff and was subsequently placed in seclusion. An hour later, the patient is calm and cooperative, so the nurse decides the patient can safely be removed from the seclusion area. What action should the nurse perform immediately after the seclusion period ends?

A. Administer an antipsychotic to prevent further episodes
B. Place a belt around the patient's pants to discourage removal
C. Help the patient reflect on the event and provide feedback
D. Complete an incident report that documents the episode

(See answers next page.)

19. B) History of asthma

Propanolol is a beta-blocker that can be prescribed for performance anxiety as well as hypertension, migraine prophylaxis, and essential tremors. Propranolol has been found to trigger severe bronchospasms, especially in patients with a history of asthma, so the nurse should contact the provider because of this contraindication. Propranolol can lower blood pressure and pulse rate; however, the current blood pressure is normal, which makes it safe to administer the medication. The patient is mildly tachycardic with a pulse of 105, but this would improve with the propanolol dose, which is a benefit, not a contraindication. Pravastatin, a statin drug, is a look-alike, sound-alike medication used to treat hyperlipidemia. It is not related to propranolol; therefore, the drug allergy would not apply to propanolol administration.

20. C) Stop the medication, then assess to see if the sleep-eating behavior continues

Zolpidem (Ambien) is a short-term treatment option for insomnia. The boxed warning associated with the medication is the risk for complex sleep behaviors such as sleep-walking, sleep-driving, and sleep-eating. For patient safety, the medication should be stopped immediately, not reduced by half, because the patient exhibits complex sleep behaviors. The patient should be reassessed to ensure the sleep behaviors resolve after the medication is stopped. Using barriers to prevent access to the kitchen creates a risk for injury and does not address the medication side effect that the patient is experiencing. Sleep-eating, regardless of the time of the day, is a safety issue because of the risk of choking and aspiration and should not be encouraged.

21. C) Help the patient reflect on the event and provide feedback

A debriefing session should be held with any patient who has been restrained or placed in seclusion immediately after the restrictive intervention is removed. The debriefing session should facilitate the patient reflecting on the events that led to the seclusion and also allow the patient an opportunity to provide feedback on their experience. Information obtained by the session can be used to identify and prevent future episodes, guide necessary treatment plan changes, and allow the patient an active voice in their treatment. If the patient is no longer demonstrating harmful behavior, an antipsychotic should not be given at this time. Belts are not permitted on the psychiatric unit because patients can use them to harm themselves or someone else. Completing an incident report that documents the situation is very important, but this would be performed after all necessary patient care is delivered.

22. A patient presents to the psychiatric emergency department with decreased level of consciousness (LOC), miosis, hypotension, and respiratory depression. The patient has a history of heroin use and is being treated by an outpatient methadone program. Which medication will the nurse immediately administer?

A. Flumazenil (Romazicon)
B. Naloxone (Narcan)
C. Lorazepam (Ativan)
D. N-acetylcysteine (NAC)

23. A patient with ombrophobia, a fear of rain, asks the nurse what they can do to help decrease their fear. Which of the following should the nurse advise the patient to do?

A. Ignore the fear and expect it to go away
B. Relocate to a drier climate to avoid rain
C. Fully immerse themselves in heavy rain
D. Occasionally expose themselves to light rain

24. A patient with a history of post-traumatic stress disorder (PTSD) is experiencing nightmares. The provider orders prazosin (Minipress) to be administered at bedtime. Prior to administering the first dose of the medication, the nurse checks the patient's:

A. Blood pressure
B. Pupil size
C. Temperature
D. Respiratory rate

25. A patient with a history of alcoholic liver disease presents for evaluation of anxiety. The patient states that they would like to try a natural supplement before taking a prescription medication. The nurse recommends:

A. Kava
B. Chamomile
C. Saint-John's-wort
D. Melatonin

(See answers next page.)

22. B) Naloxone (Narcan)

Heroin is an illicit drug that is classified as an opioid; methadone is also an opioid drug, but it can be used to treat opioid addiction. The patient is presenting with signs of an opioid overdose, which is treated with the reversal agent naloxone. The opioid overdose could be due to a heroin relapse or inappropriately taking the prescribed methadone, but both would be reversed with the administration of naloxone since they are both opioids. Flumazenil is the reversal agent for benzodiazepines. Lorazepam is not indicated because it is used for alcohol withdrawal symptoms or as a sedative; it should not be given to any patient with a decreased LOC or respiratory depression as it would worsen the symptoms. N-acetylcysteine is most commonly given for an acetaminophen overdose.

23. D) Occasionally expose themselves to light rain

When appropriate, a patient with a phobia can slowly and cautiously expose themselves to the feared object in hopes of desensitizing them to the fear over time; this is the concept that is used in exposure therapy. Ignoring the fear does not address the issue and will not help to improve the phobia. Advising the patient to relocate to a dry climate would be a drastic change and would not be a primary intervention. Fully immersing the patient in the phobia can be overwhelming and traumatic, which would worsen the phobia.

24. A) Blood pressure

Prazosin is an alpha-blocker that can be used to treat PTSD-associated nightmares as well as hypertension. Because of prazosin's blood pressure–lowering effect, the nurse should check the patient's blood pressure prior to administration; the medication should not be administered if hypotension is found. Changes in pupil size and respiratory rate are associated with other medications, such as opioids. Temperature assessment would be important when examining for neuroleptic malignant syndrome in patients who are taking antipsychotic medications.

25. B) Chamomile

Chamomile is known to have calming effects and can be safely used to treat anxiety. Kava is also known to treat anxiety symptoms; however, this supplement is contraindicated in patients with liver impairment. Saint-John's-wort is used to treat depression. Melatonin, a natural hormone that regulates the sleep–wake cycle, is used to improve sleep.

26. A patient who is taking carbamazepine (Tegretol) presents to the nurse complaining of fatigue and body aches. The nurse suspects the most serious adverse reaction associated with carbamazepine. Using the as-needed laboratoy order, which test should the nurse use to assess for the condition?

A. Urinalysis (UA)
B. Complete blood count (CBC)
C. Hepatic panel
D. Renal function panel

27. An adolescent patient presents to the clinic with a parent for a medication refill visit. The patient is prescribed amphetamine/dextroamphetamine mixed salts (Adderall XR) 20 mg once a day for the treatment of attention deficit hyperactivity disorder (ADHD). The parent reports that the patient's grades have dropped recently and that the patient sleeps more than usual. Which finding would the nurse identify as the most concerning?

A. Negative urine drug screen
B. Consistent pulse rate of 95
C. Mild dry mouth during the day
D. A 5-lb weight loss in the past year

28. A patient presents to the psychiatric emergency department with severe rigidity and hyporeflexia. The patient has a history of schizophrenia and states that they started a new medication for their condition 1 week ago but do not remember the name of the medication. Vital signs are pulse 72, blood pressure 122/84, respirations 22, and temperature 103.4°F. Laboratory results reveal an elevated serum creatine kinase level. What condition does the nurse suspect?

A. Neuroleptic malignant syndrome
B. Serotonin syndrome
C. Tardive dyskinesia
D. Drug-induced psychosis

(See answers next page.)

26. B) Complete blood count (CBC)

The use of carbamazepine (Tegretol) carries a boxed warning for agranulocytosis, a low white blood cell count, which would be seen on the patient's CBC. There is also a risk of aplastic anemia, which would also be seen on a CBC. A UA would not reveal any pertinent information since there are no known serious urinary side effects. Mild renal and/or hepatic impairment may result from any prescribed medication; however, the most serious side effect associated with this medication is agranulocytosis.

27. A) Negative urine drug screen

Patients who are prescribed amphetamine/dextroamphetamine mixed salt medications such as Adderall XR will test positive for amphetamines on a urine drug screen because of a metabolite of the medication. The absence of the medication in the drug screen combined with the recent drop in grades raises concern for noncompliance and/or possible medication diversion; therefore, the prescribing provider should be notified. The nurse should monitor the patient's blood pressure and pulse at each visit; however, the patient's pulse is normal at this time. Dry mouth is a known side effect of stimulant medications and does not require intervention. A loss of 5 lb in 1 year is not excessive or unusual for an adolescent patient.

28. A) Neuroleptic malignant syndrome

The symptoms of neuroleptic malignant syndrome include severe rigidity, hyporeflexia, extremely elevated temperature, and autonomic dysfunction. An elevated serum creatine kinase level is often seen due to the associated muscle breakdown. Neuroleptic malignant syndrome is most commonly seen with antipsychotic medications and often occurs 1 to 2 weeks after starting a new medication. Serotonin syndrome is associated with medications such as selective serotonin reuptake inhibitors (SSRIs), and symptoms include hyperreflexia, dilated pupils, muscle twitching, elevated pulse, and hypertension; an elevation in temperature or creatine kinase level would not be present. Tardive dyskinesia consists of involuntary movements such as lip smacking or eye blinking but is not associated with systemic symptoms such as vital sign changes. Drug-induced psychosis is most often seen with the use of illicit substances, with symptoms such as confusion, delusions, paranoia, and hallucinations.

29. A patient presents to the psychiatric emergency department with severe dizziness, lightheadedness, extremely blurred vision, constant nausea, vomiting, body aches, and a new onset of insomnia. The patient admits to suddenly stopping their fluoxetine (Prozac) 1 week ago because they could not afford the medication. What condition does the nurse suspect?

A. Antidepressant withdrawal syndrome
B. Serotonin syndrome
C. Neuroleptic malignant syndrome
D. Expected medication side effects

30. Which of the following statements made by a patient who is being prescribed lithium (Lithobid) indicates that further education is needed?

A. "I will increase my daily water intake."
B. "I will come to the emergency department if I develop a metallic taste."
C. "It is important to have adequate sodium intake."
D. "Elevating my feet will help with swelling."

31. A healthy young adult patient who is prescribed phenelzine (Nardil) for depression presents for a routine medication management visit. The patient reports that they do not have any complaints and that there have not been any changes to their health history. The physical examination is normal with a blood pressure of 155/92. To further assess the elevated blood pressure reading, the nurse should initially ask the patient about their:

A. Recent diet
B. Quality of sleep
C. Bowel habits
D. Work schedule

32. The nurse is assessing medication tolerance in a patient who was started on topiramate 4 weeks ago for bipolar disorder. Which of the following reported side effects would the nurse find most concerning?

A. Weight loss
B. Generalized rash
C. Evening nausea
D. Loss of appetite

(See answers next page.)

29. A) Antidepressant withdrawal syndrome

If a selective serotonin reuptake inhibitor (SSRI) is to be discontinued, the patient should be gradually weaned off the medication over the course of 2 to 4 weeks. If the medication is stopped abruptly, antidepressant withdrawal syndrome can occur. Symptoms include flu-like symptoms, dizziness, lightheadedness, nausea, sleep disturbances, and vision changes. Serotonin syndrome occurs when there is an increased, not decreased, serotonin level, and symptoms include hyperreflexia, dilated pupils, muscle twitching, elevated pulse, and hypertension. The symptoms of neuroleptic malignant syndrome include severe rigidity, hyporeflexia, extremely elevated temperature, and autonomic dysfunction; it is associated with antipsychotic medications. Expected SSRI side effects can include symptoms such as nausea and dizziness; however, these symptoms should be mild and would not develop after the medication has been stopped.

30. B) "I will come to the emergency department if I develop a metallic taste."

Because a metallic taste is an expected side effect of lithium, there is no need for the patient to present to the emergency department; the patient needs further education regarding medication expectations. Water intake should be increased because of known side effects of polydipsia and polyuria. The patient should also ensure that their sodium intake is adequate because of the risk of hyponatremia that is associated with lithium. Lastly, mild edema is a known side effect that can be relieved by elevating the feet if swelling is present in that area.

31. A) Recent diet

Phenelzine (Nardil) is a monoamine oxidase inhibitor (MAOI) used to treat depression. If foods containing tyramine are consumed while taking MAOIs, high levels of tyramine can occur, which results in concerning symptoms, particularly elevated blood pressure. Patients who are prescribed MAOIs should be advised to avoid foods that contain tyramine. To further assess the new onset of elevated blood pressure, the nurse should first ask about the patient's recent diet to assess for tyramine-containing foods, which could be the cause. Quality of sleep, bowel habits, and work schedule are all part of the general assessment but do not address the patient's current blood pressure.

32. B) Generalized rash

Stevens–Johnson syndrome is a rare, but serious, adverse reaction that can occur with topiramate therapy. The syndrome presents as a rash that spreads, worsens, and eventually develops blistered areas. Any reported rash should be immediately evaluated to rule out this potentially fatal adverse reaction. Weight loss, nausea, and loss of appetite are all expected side effects that do not require intervention.

33. The risk of a infant being born with a neurological disorder can be reduced if, before and during pregnancy, the pregnant patient takes:

A. Thiamine (vitamin B_1)
B. Folic acid (vitamin B_9)
C. Cyanocobalamin (vitamin B_{12})
D. Niacin (vitamin B_6)

34. The nurse is working in the psychiatric emergency department when an older adult patient with a history of major depression and Parkinson disease reports fever, uncontrollable shivering, cardiac arrhythmias, restlessness, and hyperreflexia. The patient reports taking paroxetine (Paxil) but is just starting on a new medication for Parkinson disease. The medication most likely to cause this drug interaction is:

A. Selegiline (Eldepryl)
B. Levodopa/carbidopa (Sinemet)
C. Cyproheptadine (Periactin)
D. Loratadine (Claritin)

35. Sexual side effects resulting from use of a selective serotonin reuptake inhibitor (SSRI) can be treated with the adjunctive medication:

A. Buspirone (Buspar)
B. Verapamil (Isoptin)
C. Bupropion (Wellbutrin)
D. Carbamazepine (Tegretol)

36. When educating the patient regarding lamotrigine (Lamictal), the nurse makes sure to discuss the rare adverse effect of Stevens–Johnson syndrome. The patient should immediately report:

A. Maculopapular rash
B. Elevated blood pressure
C. Nausea and vomiting
D. Severe headache

(See answers next page.)

33. B) Folic acid (vitamin B_9)

Folic acid is a B vitamin that is known for neuroprotection of the fetus. Although all B vitamins are vital to fetal development, folic acid is needed for neurulation, which is the process by which the neural tube is developed in utero at 3 to 4 weeks of gestation. A diet deficient in folic acid will produce neurulation defects; therefore, it is important to advise all pregnant patients to take an adequate supply of folic acid.

34. A) Selegiline (Eldepryl)

The patient is prescribed paroxetine (Paxil), which is an selective serotonin reuptake inhibitor (SSRI). Serotonin syndrome is a psychiatric emergency that occurs when an SSRI dosage is increased or when it is combined with a medication that can raise plasma levels of serotonin to toxic concentrations. Symptoms rising to the level of an emergency include fever, seizures, cardiac arrhythmias, and an altered level of consciousness. Offending medications include monoamine oxidase inhibitors (MAOIs), lithium, L-tryptophan, and others. Selegiline (Eldepryl), which is often used to treat Parkinson disease, is an MAOI. Levodopa/carbidopa, used to treat Parkinson disease, is not associated with serotonin syndrome. Cyproheptadine is an antihistamine agent that decreases serotonin levels and is often used in the treatment of serotonin syndrome. Loratadine is an antihistamine that is not associated with serotonin syndrome.

35. C) Bupropion (Wellbutrin)

Bupropion (Wellbutrin) is commonly used in the treatment of SSRI-induced sexual side effects. Buspirone (Buspar) is used in the treatment of generalized anxiety disorder and anxiety related to depression. Verapamil (Isoptin) is a calcium channel blocker that, while not officially recognized as psychotropic, is commonly used to treat some psychiatric disorders. Carbamazepine (Tegretol) is an anticonvulsant.

36. A) Maculopapular rash

Stevens–Johnson syndrome is a life-threatening adverse effect of lamotrigine use. Symptoms include a maculopapular rash that develops all over the body and begins to necrotize. This may occur when lamotrigine is titrated too rapidly or combined with valproate (Depakote). Elevated blood pressure, nausea, vomiting, and severe headache are symptoms of hypertensive crisis, which occurs when the use of monoamine oxidase inhibitors (MAOIs) is combined with the consumption of tyramine-containing foods.

37. The nurse is working with a patient who has limited resources and recommends a complementary and alternative treatment as part of their psychiatric care. A mind–body intervention that would be appropriate for this patient is:

A. Meditation
B. Massage therapy
C. Acupressure
D. Reflexology

38. The nurse is assessing an older adult patient being treated with a selective serotonin reuptake inhibitor (SSRI) for major depressive disorder who reports headache, nausea, vomiting, lethargy, and disorientation. The lab result most consistent with the suspected adverse reaction is:

A. Sodium level of 148 mEq/L
B. Sodium level of 132 mEq/L
C. Potassium level of 3.2 mmol/L
D. Potassium level of 5.5 mmol/L

39. The nurse is reviewing the chart of a 12-year-old patient with attention deficit hyperactivity disorder (ADHD). The patient has a history of a heart murmur, and the most recent EKG is abnormal. The most appropriate medication to treat the patient's ADHD is:

A. Methylphenidate (Ritalin)
B. Atomoxetine (Strattera)
C. Amphetamine (Adderall)
D. Nortriptyline (Pamelor)

(See answers next page.)

37. A) Meditation

Meditation is a technique that involves focusing on a mantra or object while practicing being present in a state of calm; it can be performed at home without the need for additional supplies or equipment. Meditation has physiological effects, such as decreasing heart and respiratory rates and blood pressure, increasing alpha brain waves, and reducing anxiety. Other examples of mind–body interventions include art therapy, yoga, dance therapy, guided imagery, biofeedback, prayer, and counseling. Massage therapy, reflexology, and acupressure are categorized as manipulative and body-based interventions; they may also require payment, which is not preferred for a patient with limited resources.

38. B) Sodium level of 132 mEq/L

Hyponatremia occurs when sodium levels fall below 135 mEq/L and includes symptoms of headache, nausea, vomiting, lethargy, and disorientation. If left untreated, it can cause seizures, coma, and death. Hyponatremia is common in older adults being treated for depression who are taking SSRIs. The syndrome of inappropriate secretion of antidiuretic hormone (SIADH) is a well-known adverse effect of SSRIs. Risk factors for the development of hyponatremia with SSRIs include older age, concomitant use of diuretics, low body weight, and lower baseline serum sodium concentration. A sodium level of 148 mEq/L indicates hypernatremia. Although the symptoms of hypernatremia are similar to those of hyponatremia, hypernatremia is not associated with the use of antidepressants or SSRIs. Antidepressants or SSRIs are also not associated with increased or decreased potassium levels.

39. B) Atomoxetine (Strattera)

Atomoxetine is a nonstimulant medication that is approved by the U.S. Food and Drug Administration for adults and children older than 6 years. It does not pose a risk of cardiac side effects and would be the safest choice for this patient. The patient's EKG is descriptive of Wolff–Parkinson–White (WPW) syndrome, a type of congenital heart condition that causes rapid heart rate or palpitations. Patients with known congenital heart disease or any type of cardiac arrhythmias should avoid use of stimulant medications because of adverse cardiac effects such as tachycardia and arrhythmias. Methylphenidate and amphetamine are stimulants that may cause adverse cardiovascular effects. Nortriptyline is a nonstimulant medication, a tricyclic antidepressant (TCA) that may be used as second- or third-line off-label treatment for ADHD. However, TCAs also have the potential to produce cardiac arrhythmias and tachycardia, which would be contraindicated for a patient with WPW syndrome.

40. A nontraditional method that helps improve brain function and cognition to further assist with building resilience is:

A. Attending weekly psychotherapy
B. Using a stimulant medication as needed
C. Joining a trauma support group
D. Engaging in regular physical exercise

41. A young adult patient calls the office and reports diarrhea, heavy sweating, goosebumps, shivering, and pupils that look slightly dilated as noted by the patient's parent. The symptoms began a few hours ago, after the patient started paroxetine (Paxil) 20 mg for depression. The nurse will:

A. Advise that these are expected side effects that usually resolve within the first 2 weeks
B. Recommend that the patient break the pills in half and only take half of a tablet for the first week
C. Tell the patient to stop the medication and make a follow-up appointment with the clinic
D. Refer the patient to the emergency department and advise the patient to stop the medication

42. A description of serotonin syndrome includes:

A. Development of headache, appetite changes, and sleep disruption that begin shortly after starting escitalopram (Lexapro) and subside and improve after a week
B. Decrease in sexual drive and libido, increase in irritability, and mild gastrointestinal upset that improves a few days after starting sertraline (Zoloft)
C. Rapid onset of agitation, confusion, muscle rigidity, fever, and elevated blood pressure hours after starting sertraline (Zoloft)
D. Increase in sweating, diarrhea, agitation, and headaches that develop 2 days after starting paroxetine (Paxil)

(See answers next page.)

40. D) Engaging in regular physical exercise
Several scientific studies indicate that physical exercise helps improve brain function and cognitive abilities, including thinking and memory. It can also help reduce the level of cortisol released from stress. Exercise as a whole can help elevate mood and calm anxiety, thereby assisting in the healing process toward recovery and building resilience. Attending weekly psychotherapy sessions, taking prescribed stimulant medications, and joining a trauma support group are forms of traditional therapy.

41. D) Refer the patient to the emergency department and advise the patient to stop the medication
The patient reports symptoms consistent with the development of serotonin syndrome, which is considered a medical emergency and requires a higher-level evaluation of symptoms. Other symptoms of serotonin syndrome include confusion, agitation, loss of muscle control, rapid heart rate, restlessness, changes in blood pressure, tremor, high fever, and seizures. The symptoms are not normal side effects and the patient should not continue taking the medication. The nurse should not suggest a change in dosage without discussing it with the prescriber. Serotonin syndrome is a serious condition that requires immediate care; this should not be postponed until a clinic appointment.

42. C) Rapid onset of agitation, confusion, muscle rigidity, fever, and elevated blood pressure hours after starting sertraline (Zoloft)
Serotonin syndrome is a medical emergency that requires prompt intervention and is a risk associated with starting selective serotonin reuptake inhibitors (SSRIs). It is characterized by a sudden onset of increased agitation, confusion, muscle rigidity, sweating, fever, extreme diarrhea, and elevated blood pressure. These issues occur shortly after starting medication with serotonergic properties; the risk of developing these issues is increased if the patient takes other drugs or supplements, such as Saint-John's-wort, that also work on serotonin. Headache, appetite change, sleep disruption, decreased libido, and mild gastrointestinal upset are all common side effects that can occur after initiating an SSRI and that generally subside after about a week. The risk of the development of side effects can be decreased by starting at a lower dosage. If symptoms are already occurring, reduce the dosage and continue monitoring the side effects and assessing for improvement.

43. A medication to reduce the risk of adverse reactions and further complications in cases of suspected opioid overdose is:

A. Naloxone
B. Naltrexone
C. Carbamazepine
D. Acamprosate

44. Boundaries, as emphasized in structural family therapy, can be defined as:

A. A negative task that is assigned when a family member is resistant
B. Problematic behaviors that are relabeled to have more positive meaning
C. Physical or psychological barriers that protect the integrity of family systems
D. Dyads that decrease stress

45. When performing family therapy, the nurse understands that the family system is a process that:

A. Involves individuals in a family working on individual problems
B. Involves family members working together
C. Is not structured on family feedback
D. Involves individuals in a family working in groups to achieve a common goal

46. Based on its mechanism of action, sertraline is a:

A. Norepinephrine and dopamine uptake inhibitor
B. Norepinephrine and serotonin–specific antidepressant
C. Serotonin and norepinephrine reuptake inhibitor
D. Selective serotonin reuptake inhibitor

47. In general, first-generation antipsychotic medications block the:

A. 5 hydroxytryptamine-2 receptor
B. Muscarinic-2 receptor
C. Alpha-1 adrenergic receptor
D. Dopamine D2 receptor

(See answers next page.)

43. A) Naloxone

Naloxone is an opioid antagonist that can rapidly reverse and quickly restore normal breathing in the case of opioid overdose, reducing the risk of further complications. Naltrexone is a mu opioid receptor antagonist used to reduce cravings and the rewarding effects of alcohol. Carbamazepine is an anticonvulsant medication that is used in the treatment of seizures and chronic neuropathic pain. Acamprosate is used for the treatment of alcohol dependence.

44. C) Physical or psychological barriers that protect the integrity of family systems

Boundaries can be defined as physical or psychological barriers that protect the integrity of family systems. Assigning a negative task to a resistant family member demonstrates paradoxical intervention. Relabeling a problematic behavior to have a more positive meaning defines reframing. Dyads that decrease stress defines triangles, found in family systems theory.

45. B) Involves family members working together

A family system is a unit structured on feedback, including a process by which all family members work together. A family system is not promoted by working on individual problems or working in separate groups. A family system is structured on feedback.

46. D) Selective serotonin reuptake inhibitor

Because sertraline possesses the capability of blocking serotonin reuptake, more of this neurotransmitter becomes available at the synapse; thus, it is a selective serotonin reuptake inhibitor. It does not inhibit the reuptake of norepinephrine and dopamine. Although it increases the neurotransmission of serotonin, it does not do the same in the case of norepinephrine; hence, it is not a norepinephrine and serotonin–specific antidepressant. It can inhibit the reuptake only of serotonin, not of norepinephrine.

47. D) Dopamine D2 receptor

First-generation antipsychotic medications perform their activities by blocking the dopamine D2 receptors. 5 hydroxytryptamine-2 receptors are serotonin receptors, which can be blocked by second-generation antipsychotic medicines, not by first-generation antipsychotic medicines. Muscarinic-2 receptors are acetylcholine receptors, which are not blocked by first-generation antipsychotic medications. First-generation antipsychotic medications also do not block the alpha-1 adrenergic receptors of epinephrine or norepinephrine.

48. A first-line treatment for Alzheimer disease is:

A. Methylphenidate
B. Donepezil
C. Carbidopa-levodopa
D. Lithium

49. A young adult patient is admitted to a psychiatric unit with a diagnosis of paranoid schizophrenia. The patient studies at a university, lives in a dormitory, and has been an excellent student. Friends describe the patient as amiable and socially active. However, for the past few months, the patient has lost interest in studies, self-care, and hygiene and has spent most of their time alone. For the past 2 days, the patient has stayed in their room and has not eaten, stating that the food has been poisoned. The patient whispers to the nurse that someone is looking at them and asking them not to share personal information. The best medication to treat the patient's condition is:

A. Haloperidol (Haldol)
B. Perphenazine (Trilafon)
C. Olanzapine (Zyprexa)
D. Loxapine (Loxitane)

50. Amphetamine (D,L) (Adderall XR) works by blocking reuptake and increasing release of:

A. Epinephrine and serotonin
B. Epinephrine and dopamine
C. Dopamine and serotonin
D. Dopamine and glutamate

51. The medication that increases the inhibitory effect of gamma-aminobutyric acid (GABA) is:

A. Alprazolam (Xanax)
B. Buspirone (Buspar)
C. Sertraline (Zoloft)
D. Vilazodone (Viibryd)

(See answers next page.)

48. B) Donepezil

Being a cholinesterase inhibitor, donepezil is part of the first-line treatment for Alzheimer disease. Methylphenidate is a psychostimulant used in the first-line treatment of attention deficit hyperactivity disorder. Carbidopa-levodopa is a combination of medicines that belongs to the first-line treatment of Parkinson disease. The mood stabilizer lithium is the first-line treatment of bipolar disorder.

49. C) Olanzapine (Zyprexa)

The patient is exhibiting all the signs and symptoms of paranoid schizophrenia: The patient is socializing less, not studying, not performing self-care, and experiencing hallucinations and delusions. This type of schizophrenia is treated with a second-generation antipsychotic drug, olanzapine (Zyprexa). Second-generation drugs can treat both the positive and the negative symptoms of schizophrenia. Haloperidol (Haldol), perphenazine (Trilafon), and loxapine (Loxitane) are all first-generation antipsychotic drugs and are used in the case of treatment of either positive or negative symptoms of schizophrenia, but not both.

50. B) Epinephrine and dopamine

Amphetamine (D,L) (Adderall XR) works by increasing both epinephrine and dopamine. This is accomplished by blocking reuptake and aiding the presynapse in releasing more of these neurotransmitters. Serotonin and glutamate, although possibly implicated in attention deficit hyperactivity disorder, are not impacted by amphetamine (D,L).

51. A) Alprazolam (Xanax)

Alprazolam (Xanax) is the medication that impacts the inhibitory effect of GABA by binding to the benzodiazepine receptor at the GABA-A ligand gate. Buspirone, vilazodone, and sertraline all affect serotonin.

52. The nurse is interviewing a patient with major depressive disorder. The patient has a medical history of epilepsy. The medication that would be contraindicated for this patient would be:

A. Fluoxetine
B. Bupropion
C. Venlafaxine
D. Aripiprazole

53. Treatment with lithium, a mood stabilizer used to treat mania in bipolar disorder, must include a(n):

A. Urine drug screen
B. Complete metabolic panel
C. Valproic acid level
D. Electroencephalogram

54. The patient will be starting a second-generation antipsychotic/mood stabilizer. The nurse explains that ongoing monitoring will include weight and height, waist circumference, blood pressure, fasting plasma glucose, and fasting lipid profile. The nurse is referring to the risk for:

A. Metabolic syndrome
B. Tardive dyskinesia (TD)
C. Extrapyramidal symptoms (EPS)
D. Stevens–Johnson syndrome

55. When educating a patient on taking a stimulant, the nurse explains that the patient may experience mydriasis if they take more than the dosage prescribed. Mydriasis is:

A. Abnormally large and dilated pupils
B. Excessive constriction of pupils
C. Amblyopia
D. Strabismus

(*See answers next page.*)

52. B) Bupropion

Bupropion (Wellbutrin) is associated with increased risk of seizures. Because of the patient's history of epilepsy, bupropion is contraindicated for treatment of the patient's depression. Fluoxetine (Prozac) and venlafaxine (Effexor) are options for treatment. Aripiprazole (Abilify) is also indicated for severe depression.

53. B) Complete metabolic panel

Lithium must be accompanied by baseline laboratory results, including complete metabolic panel, complete blood count, electrocardiogram, thyroid function tests, and liver function tests. A urine drug screen is not a standard of treatment with lithium unless substance use disorder is suspected or is being treated. Valproic acid levels are specific to treatment with sodium valproate (Depakote). An electroencephalogram would be ordered when there is concern for seizures or other neurologic conditions.

54. A) Metabolic syndrome

Metabolic syndrome can occur with all second-generation antipsychotics and includes conditions such as elevated prolactic levels, high blood pressure, high blood sugar, and high cholesterol. TD, EPS, and Stevens–Johnson syndrome are not monitored by height and weight, waist circumference, blood pressure, fasting plasma glucose, or fasting lipid profile.

55. A) Abnormally large and dilated pupils

Mydriasis is abnormally large and dilated pupils. Miosis is excessive constriction of pupils. Amblyopia (also called *lazy eye*) is poor vision that occurs in just one eye. Strabismus (also known as *crossed eyes*) presents as a misalignment of both eyes.

56. The psychiatric–mental health nurse discusses with a patient that their medication requires close monitoring because of the risk of toxcity. The nurse educates the patient on possible side effects of the medication, including polyuria, polydipsia, weight gain, metallic taste, tremor, sedation, impaired coordination, gastrointestinal distress, diarrhea, hair loss, and acne. The medication most likely prescribed is:

A. Valproate (Depakote)
B. Lamotrigine (Lamictal)
C. Lithium (Eskalith)
D. Carbamazepine (Tegretol)

57. The intervention strategy for patients with severe mental illness is based on:

A. Reduction in severity of symptoms
B. Holistic improvement of patients
C. Elimination of the impact of the disorder on daily life
D. Education of patients about their illness and recovery

58. Emergency services brings an unconscious patient to the hospital with a femoral fracture and head injuries following a motor vehicle crash. After surgery, the patient is stable. The patient's medication administration record includes alprazolam (Xanax), morphine, acetaminophen, and ibuprofen. The patient regains consciousness and asks about alprazolam, and the nurse replies that alprazolam is used:

A. For treating anxiety
B. For treating oversleeping
C. To prevent inflammation
D. To relieve pain

(*See answers next page.*)

56. C) Lithium (Eskalith)
Lithium has a narrow therapeutic window for serum drug levels, which necessitates close monitoring; it is the only medication that has acne as a possible side effect. Symptoms such as metallic taste, tremor, and significant diarrhea are more common with lithium. Valproate, lamotrigine, and carbamazepine may have some of these side effects, but acne is not one of them.

57. B) Holistic improvement of patients
According to the evidence-based approach, the best treatment strategy is planning interventions for the holistic improvement of patients. Patients learn how to cope with their mental illness more healthily when a holistic approach is considered. Therapy, which eliminates the impact of the disorder on day-to-day life, or drugs, which reduce the severity of symptoms alone, are more likely to cause relapse. Educating patients about their illness helps in raising awareness of their condition and dispels misconceptions about the recovery process, but it is not the basis for the best treatment strategy.

58. A) For treating anxiety
Alprazolam is effective in preventing anxiety attacks. It is a tranquilizer and would therefore also help the patient fall asleep. Ibuprofen is an anti-inflammatory drug. Acetaminophen is used in case of fever and pain. Morphine is used to remove the sensation of severe or mild pain.

4

Evaluation

1. A patient was started on a selective serotonin reuptake inhibitor (SSRI) for the first time 2 weeks ago. Today the nurse makes a follow-up call to the patient. What is the most important question for the nurse to ask during the call?

   A. "Have you achieved maximum benefits?"
   B. "Have most of the side effects resolved?"
   C. "Has there been any change in suicidal thoughts?"
   D. "Have your friends or family noticed positive changes?"

2. A patient with major depressive disorder is participating in interpersonal psychotherapy (IPT). The patient reports that they noticed some improvement in mood after the first two sessions. The nurse advises the patient that they will perform an evaluation to determine the outcome of the therapy once the treatment is complete. The nurse should plan to evaluate the outcomes of IPT at:

   A. 10 weeks
   B. 16 weeks
   C. 6 months
   D. 9 months

3. A patient was started on an antipsychotic medication 6 weeks ago for the treatment of schizophrenia. Based on the psychiatric evaluation, the patient was exhibiting negative schizophrenia symptoms. Which of the following symptoms should the nurse assess for?

   A. Auditory hallucinations
   B. Affective blunting
   C. Disorganized thinking
   D. Grandiose delusions

(See answers next page.)

1. C) "Has there been any change in suicidal thoughts?"

There is an increased risk for suicidal ideation after starting an SSRI that is greatest in adolescents and young adults and common during the first 2 weeks of treatment. For patient safety, it is important that the nurse assess for suicidal thoughts. Maximum benefits are not expected until 4 to 8 weeks, depending on the medication. The resolution of side effects usually does not occur until several weeks after treatment initiation. Having friends or family recognize a positive change is reassuring; however, the most important aspect to assess is suicidal ideation.

2. B) 16 weeks

IPT is a form of psychotherapy that is used to treat a variety of mental health conditions. IPT uses a very structured approach to address multiple factors, including interpersonal relationships and communication. Due to the structured nature of IPT, the active phase is limited to 12 to 16 weeks. Assessing at 10 weeks would not be optimal because this is before the end of the treatment. Waiting until 6 or 9 months to assess the outcomes would not be ideal, as the most accurate assessment would be immediately after treatment is complete, and waiting an extended period of time could also possibly create a gap in care.

3. B) Affective blunting

Negative symptoms of schizophrenia include affective blunting, lack of motivation, and anhedonia. Hallucinations, disorganized thinking, and delusions are positive symptoms of schizophrenia. It is important to differentiate between the symptoms as different medications treat different symptoms.

4. A patient presents for a follow-up visit after having medication changes last month because of side effects. The patient was previously prescribed fluphenazine (Prolixin), but the medication was discontinued last month after the patient developed signs and symptoms of tardive dyskinesia (TD). No additional medications were prescribed. What outcome would the nurse most likely find when assessing for TD during today's visit?

   A. No evidence of TD symptoms
   B. Presence of previous TD symptoms
   C. Worsening of previous TD symptoms
   D. Development of new TD symptoms

5. A patient presents to the psychiatric emergency department with severe anxiety, nausea, vomiting, and abdominal pain. The patient has a history of opioid abuse and last used 6 hours ago. The patient is enrolled in the buprenorphine/naloxone (Suboxone) treatment program and took their first dose of buprenorphine/naloxone (Suboxone) 2 hours ago. What condition does the nurse suspect?

   A. Allergic reaction to buprenorphine
   B. Opioid withdrawal symptoms
   C. Acute opioid overdose
   D. Panic attack with nausea

6. A patient presents to the clinic with a close friend for a follow-up visit. The patient has been treated for major depressive disorder for the past 6 months. The friend reports that the patient has been extremely depressed lately and has stopped answering the friend's calls. Today, the patient got a ticket for driving 100 miles per hour in a busy business district. Which evaluation tool should the nurse administer first?

   A. Columbia–Suicide Severity Rating Scale
   B. Mood Disorder Questionnaire (MDQ)
   C. General Anxiety Disorder–7 (GAD-7)
   D. Screening questions for alcohol and other drug use (CRAFFT)

7. During a follow-up call with a patient with schizoid personality disorder, the patient proudly reports that they have a new job. What question should the nurse ask about the employment to assess for improvement in the mental health symptoms?

   A. "Are you regularly attending work meetings?"
   B. "How many hours do you work each day?"
   C. "Are you allowed to communicate via email?"
   D. "Does the job offer mental health benefits?"

(See answers next page.)

4. B) Presence of previous TD symptoms

TD is a side effect associated with the use of antipsychotic medications. It is important that the causative agent, the antipsychotic, is stopped as soon as any TD symptoms are noted because oftentimes the condition becomes permanent. A complete resolution of TD symptoms would be very unlikely. Worsening symptoms and/or the development of new symptoms would be atypical; symptom progression usually stops as soon as the medication is stopped.

5. B) Opioid withdrawal symptoms

The first dose of buprenorphine/naloxone (Suboxone) should be administered at least 6 to 8 hours after the last opioid use. If the medication is administered too soon, precipitated withdrawal can occur; nausea, vomiting, and abdominal pain are withdrawal symptoms. The symptoms are not consistent with an allergic reaction or an opioid overdose. Nausea and vomiting can occur with severe anxiety; however, the clinical history is most consistent with withdrawal symptoms secondary to the recent medication administration.

6. A) Columbia–Suicide Severity Rating Scale

Distancing oneself from friends and family and reckless behavior can be signs of a number of mental health conditions, including depression. The nurse should assess for suicidal ideation first to ensure patient safety. The recent behaviors may indicate a mood disorder, but screening for a mood disorder would be performed after patient safety is assessed. Anxiety and alcohol/drug use screening can be implemented as secondary interventions if needed.

7. A) "Are you regularly attending work meetings?"

Patients with schizoid personality disorder are often seen as loners because of their aversion to social interactions and interpersonal relationships. Regularly attending work meetings is a form of socialization that would be a positive finding for this patient. The number of hours worked each day can be discussed to ensure that the patient is not working long hours, which can cause undue stress, but this is not reflective of the current disease state. The ability to communicate via email would be beneficial for this patient given their introverted nature; however, exclusive use of email for communication would be a negative finding as this could be a way of avoiding social interaction. Merely identifying if access to email communication is available does not assess for mental health progress. To facilitate access to treatment, mental health benefits would be ideal, but having benefits does not measure progress.

8. During a one-on-one session, the patient admits for the first time that they have a plan to kill the professor who gave them a failing grade. The patient describes this plan in detail, and there is evidence that the patient has started to make preparations toward making their plan a reality. Which of the following is the first action the nurse should take in response to the patient's statements?

   A. Consult social services to assist the patient with finding a different school
   B. Follow the procedure for notifying the professor of the patient's intentions
   C. Update the patient's family with this information to warrant patient admission
   D. Keep the patient away from other patients until seen by a provider

9. A patient who is being treated for trichotillomania is participating in a group activity session. To assess for positive progress with the disorder, the nurse monitors:

   A. Hygiene habits
   B. Social interactions
   C. Verbal outbursts
   D. Degree of positivity

10. A school-based meeting is scheduled for a pediatric patient with a history of oppositional defiant disorder (ODD). The patient's teachers and parents are scheduled to attend. To provide a comprehensive evaluation of the patient's progress, what additional question will the nurse ask?

    A. "Has the patient's appetite drastically increased?"
    B. "Does the patient appear to have depression?"
    C. "How many hours of the day does the patient play outside?"
    D. "How has the patient been interacting with their pets?"

(See answers next page.)

8. B) Follow the procedure for notifying the professor of the patient's intentions

Nurses have a duty to warn, which means they are obligated to notify anyone who may be in harm's way. The nurse should follow the facility's procedure for notifying the professor of the patient's intentions. Asking social services to assist the patient in finding a new school may be helpful, but the immediate concern is ensuring the safety of the intended victim. If consent is in place, the nurse can update the family with the new information; however, this would take place after the safety interventions are completed. The patient has not made threats toward anyone in the facility and is not exhibiting violent behavior, so there is no reason to keep the patient away from others at this time.

9. B) Social interactions

Trichotillomania is an impulse-control disorder that involves the irresistible urge to pull at one's own hair. Employment and social interactions are often impaired due to the patient's inability to resist the compulsion. The patient being able to control the impulse and appropriately participate in a social activity would indicate positive progress. The condition is not associated with hygiene habits and does not involve verbal outbursts. While the presence of positivity is always an encouraging finding for any mental health disorder, the presence or degree of positivity is not representative of this disease state.

10. D) "How has the patient been interacting with their pets?"

In addition to relationships with parents and teachers, evaluating ODD includes assessing for appropriate interactions with others, such as friends and pets. Inappropriate play with family pets would be a negative finding and indicate that further treatment is needed. Appetite changes are not a reflection of ODD treatment outcomes. Evaluating symptoms of depression will not evaluate the status of the patient's ODD. If depression is a concern, the parents should be asked about the symptoms of depression, not asked for the actual diagnosis. The ability to play with peers without conflict would be a positive finding, but the location of the play, inside or outside, is not a factor in evaluation.

11. A patient with a history of obsessive-compulsive disorder (OCD) presents to the mental health facility for a follow-up visit. The patient previously declined pharmacological treatments but has completed 6 months of aversion therapy and regularly attends support groups. Today, the patient reports that they feel they have made significant progress and they are able to control compulsions at this time. To directly evaluate the current status of the patient's disorder, the nurse should assess the patient's:

A. Recent levels of anxiety
B. Quality of sleep
C. Symptoms of depression
D. Number of mood swings

12. A patient with psychosis had a violent outburst and was placed in seclusion for safety. The patient has been in seclusion for the maximum time period and the nurse is performing a reassessment to determine if the patient can safely be removed from seclusion. To assess the primary element associated with the psychosis, the nurse should assess the patient's:

A. Degree of accountability
B. Current perception of reality
C. Willingness to take daily medications
D. History of prior incidents

13. An adolescent patient with a history of depression presents to the clinic with their parents. The patient's mood has significantly improved, but the patient continues to struggle with grades at school, and the parents report that the patient does not stay on task. After the appropriate screening tools are administered, the patient is diagnosed with attention deficit hyperactivity disorder (ADHD) and prescribed atomoxetine (Strattera). Two weeks after starting the medication, the nurse makes a follow-up call to the patient. What is the most important question for the nurse to ask related to this medication?

A. "What are your current grades?"
B. "Have you had a loss of appetite?"
C. "Are you taking the medication on the weekends?"
D. "Have you had any suicidal thoughts?"

(See answers next page.)

11. A) Recent levels of anxiety

OCD involves obsessions, unwanted intrusive thoughts or urges, and compulsions—repetitive activities and behaviors that are completed as an attempt to resolve the obsession. Anxiety and/or panic occurs if the patient does not perform an activity that targets the obsession. The patient reports that they are resisting compulsions at this time; however, if the patient's anxiety level is high secondary to resisting compulsions, this would indicate that the patient has not made positive progress, because increased anxiety when resisting compulsion is an expected symptom of the disorder. Being able to resist the compulsion without inducing anxiety would be a sign of positive progress. Assessing the patient's quality of sleep is part of the general mental health assessment but is not an OCD status indicator. Anxiety, not depression, is the emotional response that is associated with OCD. The number of mood swings would be a direct reflection of a mood disorder such as bipolar disorder.

12. B) Current perception of reality

The safety issue associated with psychosis is an altered perception of reality; this can include hallucinations, paranoias, and dissociations. With psychosis, the patient reacts to the reality they are experiencing, which leads to inappropriate or harmful behavior. Assessing the patient's current perception of reality identifies the patient's ability to safely return to a less restrictive environment. A lack of accountability is often seen but is not a factor that is used to determine immediate safety. If no other symptoms are present, the patient can be removed from seclusion even if they do not agree to take daily medications. In an emergency situation, medications can be administered via nonoral routes even if the patient refuses. Past incidents can help the nurse plan interventions to prevent future episodes but do not provide insight into the current situation.

13. D) "Have you had any suicidal thoughts?"

ADHD can be treated with a number of different medications, primarily oral stimulant medications. Atomoxetine (Strattera) is a nonstimulant medication that selectively inhibits norepinephrine reuptake. Due to the mechanism of action, patients, particularly adolescents and young adults, are at risk for suicidal ideation during the initial treatment period. It is important that the nurse assess the patient for suicidal thoughts. Current grades are assessed to help determine treatment effectiveness, but this would come after ensuring patient safety by screening for suicidal thoughts. A mild loss of appetite is a known side effect of the medication, so assessing this element would be a lower priority. The nurse should discuss the medication schedule to ensure that it is being taken as prescribed, but only after all urgent issues are addressed.

14. One month after starting treatment for bulimia nervosa, the patient presents to the mental health facility for a reassessment. The patient is extremely positive and reports that everything is going well. The patient states that they no longer have any bulimic activity and all symptoms have resolved. The nurse is suspicious of the rapid resolution. Which of the following would indicate that the patient may still be experiencing symptoms of the condition?

A. The patient has had six sexual partners since starting treatment
B. The patient has been undergoing extensive dental work
C. The patient has changed their friend group at school
D. The patient disclosed their diagnosis to their intimate partner

15. The nurse is attempting to administer evening medications to a patient admitted with a substance use disorder. Included in the evening medications is a new medication that has been prescribed for insomnia. After learning of the new medication, the patient states that they do not want to take the medication until they are provided with more information about it. How should the nurse respond to the patient's statement?

A. Instruct the patient to take the medication now and state that more information may be provided at a later time
B. Hold the medication, document the interaction, and provide printed information on the medication
C. Discontinue the medication and update the prescribing provider of the change in the treatment plan
D. Tell the patient that this is a new medication and that there is no information that can be provided at this time

16. The spouse of a patient with bipolar disorder calls the office and reports that they believe the patient is manic. The patient has been hyperactive and talking about wanting to have a cosmetic procedure. Which of the following would be the best question for the nurse to ask when assessing for acute mania?

A. "How many times has your spouse initiated sexual intercourse with you?"
B. "Has the patient had excessive spending lately?"
C. "When did the abnormal behavior initially start?"
D. "Did the patient admit that they were manic?"

(See answers next page.)

14. A) The patient has had six sexual partners since starting treatment
Secondary symptoms of bulimia nervosa include hypersexual activity. The patient having six sexual partners in the past month should be further evaluated, as this could be a sign that the bulimia symptoms have not resolved as reported. Dental work may be needed to correct dental issues associated with purging behaviors. Changing friend groups is not a behavior that is directly related to bulimia. Disclosing the diagnosis to an intimate partner is a positive finding that would not be concerning.

15. B) Hold the medication, document the interaction, and provide printed information on the medication
In this nonemergency interaction, the patient should be provided information on the medication as requested by the patient because this is a component of informed consent. Requiring the patient to take the medication before providing the requested information would violate the standards of informed consent. The medication should only be discontinued with an order from a provider; the patient requesting medication information is not a reason to discontinue the medication immediately. Medication information is available for all medications that can be prescribed, including new medications.

16. C) "When did the abnormal behavior initially start?"
In order for the patient to meet the criteria for a manic episode, the symptoms must be present for at least 1 week. Having a single activity or behavior does not meet the criteria for mania. Hypersexual activity and excessive spending are common during a manic episode but are not diagnostic. The patient stating that they are manic does not automatically deem the behavior as mania, and denying mania does not exclude the diagnosis.

17. During a follow-up visit, a patient who has been treated with fluoxetine (Prozac) for depression for 1 year expresses concern over the sexual side effects they are still experiencing. Despite trying previously recommended nonpharmacological methods, the patient is experiencing significant erectile dysfunction (ED). Which of the following recommendations should the nurse make?

    A. Reduce the medication dose by 50% for 3 months
    B. Consult a urologist for ED treatment
    C. Set new sexual expectations for their relationship
    D. Explore their sexual identity with their therapist

18. The nurse is performing a home visit for a young adult with a history of bipolar disorder. The patient lives alone in an apartment on a college campus and is currently stable. Six months ago, the patient had an episode of mania. Their behavior became erratic and violent, which led to their neighbors calling the police. The patient could not provide any rational information and was hostile with the police. As a result, the police initially took the patient to the police station before transferring the patient to the hospital for evaluation. To facilitate long-term safety and stability, which of the following would the nurse suggest?

    A. Place a sign on the apartment's front door that states that the patient has bipolar disorder
    B. Disclose the mental health diagnosis to the closest neighbors
    C. Add the patient's health history to the lease agreement
    D. Obtain a medical alert bracelet and wear it at all times

19. The nurse working with the assertive community treatment team makes a home visit for a patient with a pedophilic disorder. The patient has completed 6 months of cognitive behavioral therapy and is compliant with all prescribed medications. Which statement by the patient requires further investigation by the nurse?

    A. "I decided to become a vegetarian as part of my lifestyle changes."
    B. "I got a full-time job as a janitor at the local middle school."
    C. "I shared details of my diagnosis with a few of my friends."
    D. "I participate in online support groups instead of in-person groups."

(See answers next page.)

17. B) Consult a urologist for ED treatment

Sexual side effects, including ED, are common with the use of selective serotonin reuptake inhibitors (SSRIs) such as fluoxetine. Some improvement, and possible resolution, can be seen after the initial treatment period; however, symptoms that are present after 1 year of treatment would not be expected to resolve. ED associated with SSRI use can be treated with ED medications such as tadalafil (Cialis) and sildenafil (Viagra). The patient should consult with a urologist for ED treatment. If the patient's mental health condition is well controlled on the current medication, the dose of the medication should not be changed; if a change in the dose is needed, the change should be ordered by the provider. The nurse would not be acting as a patient advocate if they advised the patient to lower their expectations before exploring all possible resolutions. The patient has expressed dissatisfaction with their current sexual performance due to the medication; there is no indication that the symptoms are related to questions around sexual identity.

18. D) Obtain a medical alert bracelet and wear it at all times

Certain medical and mental health conditions can manifest as symptoms that are concerning to others; violence is such a symptom. If background information is not available, police officers will respond as they would with any other person who demonstrates violent behavior. Because the patient may not be able to appropriately communicate during a crisis, the nurse should suggest methods that would facilitate safe transfer to a mental health facility should a future episode arise. A medical alert bracelet is a simple and discreet way of ensuring information about the patient's mental health condition is available in a crisis. Interventions such as telling the patient to place a sign on their door or to disclose their private health information to their neighbors breaches the patient's confidentiality. While there may be an option to add medical information to the patient's profile in the leasing office, this would not be useful in the event of a crisis that is outside of office hours; it would also breach the patient's confidentiality.

19. B) "I got a full-time job as a janitor at the local middle school."

Pedophilic disorders involve strong urges or compulsive behavior of a sexual nature that involves children. A primary goal of treatment is to learn to resist the urges and compulsions. Patients should avoid placing themselves in situations that would trigger the behavior; therefore, working around children would not be an appropriate job for this patient. There are no dietary factors related to pedophila treatment outcomes. Making the decision to share information about the mental health condition indicates that the patient is accepting of their diagnosis. Online support groups are an acceptable option and can be especially beneficial for those who are not comfortable discussing their condition face-to-face.

20. The nurse is conducting a follow-up call with a patient who is prescribed lithium (Lithobid) for bipolar bisorder. The patient's most recent lithium level is 0.5 mEq/L. What question would be important for the nurse to ask in regard to the laboratory finding?

A. "Have you experienced any symptoms such as nausea, vomiting, diarrhea, or abdominal pain?"

B. "Can you tell me how you have been taking the medication over the past month?"

C. "How much vitamin C have you included in your diet in the past 1 to 2 weeks?"

D. "Are you storing the medication in a cool environment such as the refrigerator?"

21. A patient who is being treated for alcohol use disorder presents to the clinic for a scheduled follow-up appointment. During the previous visit, the patient stated that they intended to start Alcoholics Anonymous (AA) meetings the following week. Today, the patient reports that they did not start the meetings because they decided to reconsider if their condition is severe enough to warrant major changes. Based on this information, what would be the correct interpretation of the patient's progress by the nurse?

A. The patient no longer believes they have a substance use problem

B. The patient has not made any progress but has not declined

C. Deeply considering the intervention is a positive sign

D. The patient has regressed in their progress

22. A patient presents to the psychiatric emergency department with a history of bipolar disorder. The patient reports occasional vomiting, abdominal pain, dry mouth, some dizziness, and weakness. The lithium level that would be consistent with these symptoms is:

A. 0.8 mEq/L

B. 1.4 mEq/L

C. 2.5 mEq/L

D. 0.3 mEq/L

(See answers next page.)

20. B) "Can you tell me how you have been taking the medication over the past month?"

The therapeutic window for a lithium level is 0.8 to 1.2 mEq/L; therefore, the current laboratory result is subtherapeutic. The nurse would first ensure that the patient is taking the medication as prescribed by asking how they have been taking the medication. Symptoms such as nausea, diarrhea, and abdominal pain are associated with a high lithium level (i.e., lithium toxicity). Vitamin C does not alter lithium levels. Storing the medication in a cool environment, such as a refrigerator, is not needed to maintain the potency of the medication; it can be safely stored at room temperature.

21. D) The patient has regressed in their progress

When evaluating a patient with a history of substance use, it is important to assess the stage of change the patient is currently in. During the previous visit, the patient was in the preparation stage based on their intent to take action by starting AA meetings. Questioning if change is needed is consistent with the contemplation stage, indicating that the patient has regressed in the recovery process. The patient is currently contemplating the need for change to address the disorder; they have not denied that they have a substance use problem. The patient has reverted to a previous stage of change, which is not a neutral finding. Deeply considering change at this time is not a positive sign since the patient was previously in the preparation stage.

22. C) 2.5 mEq/L

The patient is exhibiting mild to moderate intoxication of lithium, which presents with symptoms of vomiting, abdominal pain, dry mouth, ataxia, dizziness, slurred speech, nystagmus, lethargy or excitement, and muscle weakness. An elevated lithium level of 2.5 mEq/L would correlate with the symptoms. Lithium levels of 0.8 mEq/L and 1.4 mEq/L are both therapeutic levels for bipolar maintenance. A level of 0.3 mEq/L would be subtherapeutic and would not result in the patient's current symptoms.

23. A patient presents to the psychiatric emergency department with a history of bipolar disorder. The patient reports dizziness and abdominal pain. The patient's lithium level is 1.8 mEq/L. Other symptoms the nurse expects to see include:

A. Vomiting and dry mouth
B. Profuse sweating and weight loss
C. Blurred vision and syncope
D. Lethargy and weight gain

24. Spina bifida is a common defect found in neonates exposed during the first trimester to:

A. Carbamazepine (Tegretol)
B. Folic acid (Folacin)
C. Paroxetine (Paxil)
D. Lamotrigine (Lamictal)

25. Complications occurring within days of beginning antipsychotic treatment can include moderate to severe elevation in temperature, muscle rigidity, altered consciousness, and autonomic instability, which are most likely related to:

A. Serotonin syndrome
B. Neuroleptic malignant syndrome
C. Anticholinergic syndrome
D. Malignant hyperthermia

26. According to the Patient's Bill of Rights, the patient right that relates to protection of a patient's health information is the right to:

A. Have every consideration of privacy
B. Expect that all communication about care will be treated as confidential
C. Receive high-quality treatment
D. Know the identity of all healthcare staff involved in the patient's care

(*See answers next page.*)

23. A) Vomiting and dry mouth

Mild to moderate lithium toxicity is seen in patients with lithium levels between 1.5 and 2.0 mEq/L. Signs of mild to moderate lithium toxicity include vomiting, abdominal pain, dry mouth, ataxia, dizziness, slurred speech, nystagmus, lethargy or excitement, and muscle weakness. Profuse sweating and weight loss are symptoms of hyperthyroidism. Blurred vision and syncope are symptoms of moderate to severe lithium toxicity. Lethargy and weight gain are symptoms of hypothyroidism.

24. A) Carbamazepine (Tegretol)

Carbamazepine is associated with neural tube defects, such as spina bifida. Folic acid is used to protect the neural development of a fetus, and all pregnant patients should be instructed to take folic acid. Although paroxetine is a teratogen, it does not cause neural tube defects, but it is associated with cardiac malformations. Lamotrigine is associated with cleft palate.

25. B) Neuroleptic malignant syndrome

Neuroleptic malignant syndrome typically occurs within days after exposure to an antipsychotic, with core symptoms including severe muscle rigidity, altered consciousness, elevated temperature, and autonomic dysregulation. Although muscle rigidity is a possible indication of serotonin syndrome, symptoms of this condition usually occur within several hours of taking a new drug or increasing a dosage. Antipsychotics may cause anticholinergic syndrome; however, symptoms of this condition include flushing, dry mucous membranes, hypertension, tachycardia, and urinary retention. Malignant hyperthermia can occur when the patient is exposed to drugs usually used for anesthesia, and symptoms include severe muscle rigidity, shallow and rapid breathing, tachycardia, arrhythmia, dangerously high body temperature, and excessive sweating.

26. B) Expect that all communication about care will be treated as confidential

The right to expect that all communication and records pertaining to a patient's care will be treated as confidential is specific to protection of a patient's health information. The right to every consideration of privacy, the right to quality treatment, and the right to know the identity of all healthcare staff involved in a patient's care are included in the Patient's Bill of Rights but do not pertain to protection of a patient's health information.

27. A 15-year-old patient is seen in the psychiatric emergency department with reports of uncontrolled shivering, tremors, and diarrhea. The patient recently started fluoxetine (Prozac) for depression. After the patient experienced anxiety earlier in the day, the patient's parent gave the patient an over-the-counter supplement to help calm the patient down. The nurse suspects that the patient's symptoms are caused by the supplement:

A. Saint-John's-wort
B. Valerian root
C. Chamomile extract
D. Passionflower

(See answers next page.)

27. A) Saint-John's-wort

The patient is displaying signs and symptoms of serotonin syndrome. Although many over-the-counter supplements may be used to treat anxiety, only Saint-John's-wort is contraindicated for use with antidepressants such as selective serotonin reuptake inhibitors (SSRIs) and monoamine oxidase inhibitors (MAOIs). Fluoxetine is a common SSRI used in the treatment of depression in children and is approved by the U.S. Food and Drug Administration for patients age 8 years and older. Along with its sedative and anxiolytic effects, Saint-John's-wort is used for its antidepressant effects and acts by increasing levels of serotonin; therefore, it is contraindicated with concomitant use of other medications that increase serotonin.

Part II

Practice Examination and Answers With Rationales

5

Practice Examination

1. An adolescent patient visits the mental health clinic. The patient reports experiencing severe depression, and the mental state of the patient is adversely affecting the family. The patient acknowledges the parents' struggle to give the patient a better life. The nurse suggests that the patient:

   A. Join family dinners even if just to sit at the dinner table
   B. Stop engaging in family activities when they are sad
   C. Skip antidepressant medication when they start feeling better
   D. Refrain from sharing their feelings with family members

2. The cause of a patient's clinical depression is conflict with their spouse. The patient is advised to work on communication with their spouse to improve their relationship. This approach is part of the therapy known as:

   A. Aversion
   B. Behavioral
   C. Interpersonal
   D. Psychoanalytic

3. A patient is asked to monitor heart rate, respiratory rate, and blood pressure whenever the patient has episodes of major depression. This monitoring is an example of which type of therapy?

   A. Aversion
   B. Interpersonal
   C. Modeling
   D. Biofeedback

4. The treatment plan for a patient with generalized anxiety disorder recommends a complementary treatment. An example of a complementary therapy would be:

   A. Systematic desensitization/exposure therapy
   B. Electroconvulsive therapy
   C. Transcranial magnetic stimulation
   D. Meditation

5. The nurse is treating an older adult patient who wants to take only "natural medicine." The patient is showing difficulty with memory and cognitive performance. A natural supplement associated with improving cognition is:

   A. Valerian

   B. Melatonin

   C. Ginkgo biloba

   D. Omega-3 fatty acids

6. A young adult patient with marked functional decline for the past 10 months has been diagnosed with schizophrenia and prescribed aripiprazole (Abilify). The patient has elevated hemoglobin A1C, hyperlipidemia, and weight gain. The patient presents with active auditory hallucinations (command type) and persecutory delusions. The priority of the assessment should be:

   A. Medication compliance

   B. Side effects of aripiprazole

   C. Focus on reality testing

   D. Suicidal behavior

7. The nurse is taking care of a newly pregnant patient with schizophrenia. The patient wants to continue the pregnancy, but the family prefers that the patient have an abortion. To promote the safety of the fetus, the patient's antipsychotic medication would need to be reduced, putting the patient at risk of exacerbating the psychiatric illness. Furthermore, the question has been raised as to whether the patient can safely care for the baby. Eventually, the patient decides to carry the pregnancy to term. The ethical principle that allows this decision is:

   A. Autonomy

   B. Beneficence

   C. Fidelity

   D. Veracity

8. The nurse is preparing to administer a medication to a patient. When the nurse enters the room, the patient shows anxiety. The nurse calms the patient, and only when the patient feels comfortable does the nurse administer the prescribed drug. This is an example of:

   A. Beneficence

   B. Justice

   C. Autonomy

   D. Veracity

9. A 23-year-old patient is being treated for mania and has been prescribed valproic acid (Depakote). The patient reports sudden loss of appetite, extreme fatigue, and nausea. The urine is dark, and the patient is jaundiced. There are no other complaints or previous contributing history. Laboratory results are normal except for moderately elevated liver function tests. Based on the patient history, a possible diagnosis is:

A. Gallbladder disease
B. Drug-induced liver injury
C. Biliary cirrhosis
D. Blood dyscrasia

10. A nurse has a deeply religious belief system and believes everyone needs the support of a church for their survival. The nurse is working with an agnostic patient. In the therapeutic relationship with the patient, the nurse understands the differences in the beliefs and values held between them. The nurse continues to serve the patient well, and this behavior of the nurse is a result of:

A. Self-awareness
B. Values
C. Beliefs
D. Supervision

11. A patient with a clinical history of attention deficit hyperactivity disorder (ADHD) is diagnosed with Tourette syndrome. The medication that would be most appropriate for this patient would be:

A. Amphetamine (D)
B. Clonidine
C. Methylphenidate (D,L)
D. Diazepam

12. A patient who does shift work presents to the clinic to report fatigue and drowsiness for the past 3 months that is affecting job performance. A medication that is commonly used to treat this condition is:

A. Armodafinil
B. Clomipramine
C. Desipramine
D. Diazepam

13. A 22-year-old patient is admitted to a hospital for treatment for schizophrenia and is prescribed the antipsychotic clozapine. Within the first week of treatment, the patient shows signs of spasms, muscle stiffness, dry mouth, and cramping. This is immediately reported and treated with an anticholinergic drug. The nurse suspects that the patient:

 A. Had an overdose of antipsychotics
 B. Was experiencing extrapyramidal symptoms
 C. Has developed myocarditis
 D. Needs to change the medication

14. A patient with hypertension visits the clinic and reports blisters along with reddish and purplish spots accompanied by fever. The clinical history of the patient involves alcohol addiction, excessive sleepiness, and bipolar depression. The nurse should ask if the patient takes:

 A. Armodafinil
 B. Carbamazepine
 C. Chlordiazepoxide
 D. Clonidine

15. Antidepressants resolve the depressive episodes associated with deficiency of transmission of monoamine neurotransmitters by:

 A. Stimulating the effects of gamma-aminobutyric acid (GABA)
 B. Stimulating the reuptake of norepinephrine
 C. Stimulating the reuptake of dopamine
 D. Blocking the reuptake of serotonin

16. The most high-risk medication used in the treatment of acute mania in bipolar disorder is:

 A. Lurasidone (Latuda)
 B. Cariprazine (Vraylar)
 C. Lithium (Lithobid)
 D. Lamotrigine (Lamictal)

17. The nurse should maintain confidentiality when the patient:

 A. Is suicidal and can cause self-harm
 B. Reports a domestic violence situation
 C. Is not harmful to themself or others
 D. Expresses intent to harm a known person

18. To promote a safe space for communication in group therapy, the nurse should ask the members of the group to:

A. Put their phones on silent mode during the session
B. Switch their phones off completely during the session
C. Avoid speaking to each other after the session
D. Not talk about their concerns outside the group

19. The statement that best describes how self-determination impacts treatment of mental health patients is:

A. Self-determination allows patients to understand their rights while obtaining mental health treatment
B. Promoting self-determination in a patient with mental illness can result in irrational decision-making with poor outcomes
C. Patients who feel autonomous and independent are more receptive to treatment and have more successful outcomes
D. When patients feel their rights are being upheld and they can choose care options, they most often will make informed decisions

20. During evaluation, a patient with mental illness becomes agitated and begins to show aggressive behavior. To ensure the patient's right to a least-restrictive environment is met, the nurse will first:

A. Refer the patient to the psychiatrist for further evaluation
B. Attempt to de-escalate the situation by removing stimulation
C. Ask a family member or guardian for permission to restrain the patient
D. Administer diazepam based on patient level of anxiety and aggression

21. A 16-year-old patient visits the mental health facility with their parents. The parents report that the patient has an older sibling who has bipolar I disorder. The patient is at risk for which disorder?

A. Schizotypal personality
B. Narcissistic personality
C. Cyclothymic
D. Conduct

22. An older adult patient visits the office accompanied by two people. Before starting the interviewing process, to maintain the patient's confidentiality, the nurse should first:

A. Avoid asking about the relationship between the two people and the patient
B. Ask the two people accompanying the patient to wait outside the room
C. Ask the patient's permission to allow the two people to stay in the room
D. Discuss the patient's issues in front of the other two people

23. A patient reports to the nurse that they avoid places that require standing in line or staying in an enclosed place due to feelings that they could be trapped. The patient also experiences panic whenever a situation becomes a bit difficult. The nurse suspects:

A. Major depressive disorder
B. Kleptomania
C. Agoraphobia
D. Hoarding disorder

24. An adult patient is brought to the mental health facility by their parents. The patient tells the nurse about having magical powers to make dead people alive by touching them. The nurse describes this as what type of delusion?

A. Erotomanic
B. Nihilistic
C. Grandiose
D. Persecutory

25. A 77-year-old patient visits the mental health facility with their adult son. The son says that the patient has recently spent some days in the ICU after experiencing a stroke. After being discharged from the hospital, the patient talks constantly about the fear of dying. In the clinical interview, the nurse should:

A. Start by fully addressing the new onset of the fear of dying
B. Address the son and the patient by their first names in a friendly manner
C. Ask the son to stay for the interview because of the patient's age
D. Ask sensitive questions only when the patient is alone

26. A patient visits the mental health facility. The clinical record shows that the patient visited frequently a year ago for depression due to the death of their youngest child. During the interview, the patient states that the therapies were of little effect and that they still experience difficulty in managing everyday activities. The patient reports ongoing insomnia for 2 months and the inability to take care of their other children. The patient expresses self-blame throughout the interview for the loss of the youngest child. The nurse should:

A. Discuss a personal experience that involves grief and loss to make the patient comfortable
B. Tell the patient that their child is with God now, which should bring comfort
C. Educate the patient regarding the normal grief process and how the patient can get on track
D. Express that it is difficult to understand the feelings of the patient at present

27. The nurse finds that a patient has experienced a hypomanic episode and two major depressive episodes. The patient has never experienced a manic episode. According to the given diagnostic criteria, the nurse suspects that the patient has the disorder known as:

A. Bipolar II
B. Bipolar I
C. Panic
D. Cyclothymic

28. A patient reports temper outbursts occurring over the course of a year. The anger is expressed verbally and is recurrent (3 to 4 times per week). The nurse suspects the disorder called:

A. Disruptive mood dysregulation
B. Persistent depressive
C. Oppositional defiant
D. Intermittent explosive

29. A patient feels sudden trembling, sweating, and increased heart rate, accompanied by intense fear. The nurse understands the symptoms are consistent with the diagnostic criteria for the disorder called:

A. Panic
B. Bipolar
C. Hoarding
D. Excoriation

30. A nurse is performing a clinical interview with a patient with depression. To know whether the patient is experiencing impaired coping, the nurse should ask if the:

A. Patient feels rejected and not good enough
B. Patient feels angry at a greater power
C. Patient's sexual pattern has changed
D. Patient's problem-solving skills have deteriorated

31. The nurse is working with a family that reports dysfunctional communication with each other. While interviewing the family members to determine if they manipulate each other, the nurse should ask if they:

A. Grant each other's requests only after keeping some strings attached
B. Bring up irrelevant issues when a family member is discussing a problem
C. Accuse each other of responsibility for the issues occurring in the family
D. Pretend to be well-meaning to maintain peace within the family

32. A patient states that their father passed away a week ago. The first response by the nurse is to:

A. Ask about the patient's feelings regarding the loss
B. State that the loss is upsetting and ask the patient to share further
C. Express that they are sorry for the loss and show interest in knowing more
D. Reassure the patient that this phase will soon pass

33. The nurse is interviewing a patient with suicidal ideation. To know if the patient is suffering from hopelessness, the nurse should ask if the patient:

A. Faces issues regarding problem-solving
B. Has become addicted to drugs or alcohol
C. Feels like a burden on others
D. Has developed a feeling of isolation

34. A patient with hearing loss in one ear visits with the nurse after reporting symptoms of depression. During the clinical interview, the nurse will:

A. Face the patient in good lighting
B. Speak at a higher volume than usual
C. Look down at papers while interviewing
D. Explain the instructions verbally before closing

35. During a follow-up assessment, a patient who is prescribed sertraline (Zoloft) 100 mg per day for obsessive-compulsive disorder tendencies reports taking Saint-John's-wort to help with their anxiety-related depression. Upon learning this information, the nurse will:

A. Provide education on the safe use of herbal supplements and proper dosages
B. Have the patient discontinue sertraline while taking Saint-John's-wort
C. Explain that Saint-John's-wort is known to worsen mental health symptoms
D. Advise against Saint-John's-wort due to interactions with the prescribed medication

36. At a follow-up visit with a patient diagnosed with schizophrenia who is taking risperidone (Risperdal), it is discovered that the patient has gained 11.5 lb (5.2 kg). To address the weight gain associated with the medication, the nurse suggests:

A. Referral to a weight-loss specialist for further treatment
B. Stopping the medication until the next appointment
C. Adding a combination herbal supplement for weight reduction
D. Implementing the DASH diet and monthly monitoring sessions

37. A patient with anger management issues visits the mental health facility. During the interview, it is revealed that the patient uses an herb given by a traditional healer of their culture. The patient believes the herb is calming during times of anger and aggression. The nurse knows that this herb causes cognitive impairment. The nurse will:

   A. Encourage the patient to continue using the herb but only if also taking a prescribed medication
   B. Advise the patient that the facility will not provide care while they are using the herb
   C. Educate the patient regarding the serious side effects and demand that they stop the herb immediately
   D. Negotiate with the patient to reduce herb usage while discussing a possible trial of prescribed medication

38. A 5-year-old patient visits the clinic. The patient's parents report that the patient is restless and impulsive and has difficulty doing multiple tasks at one time. Appropriate treatment options include:

   A. Cognitive behavioral therapy
   B. Home school or virtual learning
   C. Honey and white rice in the diet
   D. Donepezil for the patient's symptoms

39. While collecting the history of a new patient, the nurse discovers that the patient belongs to a different cultural background than the nurse. During the interview, the nurse notices that the patient suddenly seems uncomfortable and becomes reluctant to answer questions. The patient abruptly stands up and accuses the nurse of being harsh and disrespectful. Fearing unintentionally causing the patient pain, the nurse:

   A. Pauses collecting the history and politely asks the patient which behavior was offensive
   B. Offers reassurance to the patient and moves on to the next question
   C. Asks another nurse to complete the interview
   D. Refrains from asking questions about the patient's culture and practices

40. A 22-year-old patient is brought to the emergency department by law enforcement after an explosive outburst at a local bar, where the patient physically assaulted a customer, causing injuries to the customer as well as property damage. The officers report that witnesses say the patient was laughing and having fun when they suddenly became enraged and attacked the another person. The patient is now combative, screaming obscenities, and threatening both officers and health professionals. The action the nurse would take first to address the emergency is:

A. Ask the officers to place the patient in handcuffs until an assessment can be performed
B. Request that hospital security accompany the nurse into the patient interview
C. Restrain the patient in the hospital bed until they can be evaluated by the provider
D. Contact a family member to determine the medications the patient takes at home

41. The nurse is evaluating an adult male patient brought in after experiencing a psychotic episode at home. The patient appears calm and oriented to people, place, and time. Suddenly the patient becomes agitated, is talking to himself, and begins pacing back and forth, moving closer and closer to the nurse. The nurse, feeling unsafe, will immediately:

A. Calmly speak to the patient in a slow manner, asking what has happened to upset him
B. Softly ask the patient to have a seat and engage them in conversation on how he is feeling
C. Leave the room for safety and have another provider continue the evaluation
D. Step away from the patient and call for security to be present for the rest of the assessment

42. A patient admitted from the emergency department (ED) for treatment of alcohol dependence syndrome suddenly becomes disoriented and demonstrates paranoid behaviors. When questioned, the patient states that "the voice" is telling them to set the bed on fire so they can get away and not have their "brain probed." An appropriate action by the nurse would be to:

A. Request an order for physical restraints from the ED provider
B. Provide the patient with education on weaning from alcohol
C. Administer naloxone due to suspected alcohol intoxication
D. Collect a blood specimen from the patient for thiamine level

43. A patient is brought to the mental health facility with court orders for involuntary commitment after attempting to murder their life partner, claiming that voices were instructing them to rid the earth of their partner's "kind." When the patient learns of the commitment, they become enraged and aggressive toward the staff while stating, "I'm not staying." The nurse will:

A. Continue the process to admit the patient according to the court order
B. Request a second opinion from another provider before admitting the patient
C. Discuss alternatives to the involuntary commitment with the patient
D. Deny the involuntary commitment until the patient is calmer

44. A 15-year-old patient is undergoing treatment for substance use disorder and intermittent explosive disorder. The parents are going through a hostile divorce, which has resulted in the mother and children relocating to an apartment in a new school district. These changes have resulted in a crisis that has affected the patient's recovery. The patient reports that their mother imposes punitive measures for infractions. Based on this information, the nurse determines that:

A. The patient and the family can benefit from functional family therapy
B. The patient's mother should complete parenting classes before participating in treatment
C. Stopping the patient's drug use will resolve the crisis and correct the dysfunction at home
D. The patient should live with their father temporarily to give the mother some time away from the patient

45. During assessment of a patient diagnosed with depression, the patient reports drinking more alcohol lately, describing consumption of six to eight beers at least 4 out of 7 days. To further assess the severity of the alcohol use, the nurse will choose the screening tool called:

A. CAGE
B. AUDIT
C. T-ACE
D. SBIRT

46. A child is now able to sort objects according to characteristics such as shape, type, color, size, and whether objects are broken and can be fixed. The child can put things in order based on characteristics or criteria. The child can choose between options but is unable to use deductive reasoning or logic or draw conclusions. According to Piaget, this cognitive ability indicates that the child is in the stage called:

A. Formal operational
B. Concrete operational
C. Preoperational
D. Sensorimotor

47. While working with a new patient admitted for bipolar disorder, the nurse smells alcohol and notes that the patient appears distracted and has a somewhat disheveled appearance. The initial assessment tool used by the nurse is:

A. CAGE
B. AUDIT
C. T-ACE
D. SBIRT

48. During the first session with a patient to review the treatment plan, the nurse and the patient discuss the risks and benefits of various options for psychotropic medications, the treatment plan goals, and the alterations in the treatment plan. The nurse is nurturing the therapeutic alliance through:

A. Setting limits or boundaries
B. Shared decision-making
C. Self-identification as the expert
D. Creating a safety plan

49. The excitatory neurotransmitter involved in kindling, seizure disorders, and possible bipolar disorder is:

A. Glutamate
B. Gamma-aminobutyric acid (GABA)
C. Acetylcholine
D. Glycine

50. The nurse is planning an educational session on substance use for a local shelter. After providing a lecture on the topic, the nurse plans to supply the patients with reference material to keep for the future. Which of the following is the most important factor for the nurse to consider when selecting the reference material?

A. Average age of the attendees
B. Length of reference material
C. Staff members' preference
D. Literacy level of reference material

51. Patients who use antipsychotic medications and are poor metabolizers of *CYP2D6* are at risk for:

A. Inadequate dosing
B. Antipsychotic-induced extrapyramidal symptoms
C. Loss of efficacy
D. Gene–drug interactions

52. A Spanish-speaking patient is admitted to the unit with depression. The patient is withdrawn and does not participate in activities. Which of the following would be a priority assessment to ensure appropriate interventions are planned?

A. Gender identity
B. Communication
C. Risk factors
D. Citizenship

53. The nurse is preparing to administer lithium (Lithobid) for the first time to a young adult female patient. Which of the following would be important for the nurse to ask prior to administration of the medication?

A. "Are you using any type of birth control at this time?"
B. "When was the last time you had an eye exam?"
C. "Do you ever take acetaminophen (Tylenol) for pain?"
D. "Have you been diagnosed with sleepwalking in the past?"

54. The nurse is providing discharge instructions to a patient who has been prescribed lamotrigine (Lamictal) for the first time. The patient states that they do not want to take the medication because it is for seizures. The nurse explains to the patient that lamotrigine is also used to improve:

A. Mood
B. Attention span
C. Sleep
D. Tremors

55. The nurse is administering a benzodiazepine, alprazolam (Xanax), to a patient newly diagnosed with generalized anxiety disorder. Which of the following reflects appropriate understanding of this treatment by the nurse?

A. The dose of the medication will be consistently increased over the next 3 to 6 months to reach the target dose
B. Long-term use of alprazolam is an appropriate substitute for selective serotonin reuptake inhibitors (SSRIs)
C. Because of the associated abuse potential, the patient will need intermittent benzodiazepine blood tests
D. The nurse should ask about other inventions that were tried prior to administering the alprazolam

56. While administering a scheduled dose of lithium (Lithobid) to a patient, the patient asks the nurse how the medication works to improve their condition. Which of the following would be an appropriate response by the nurse?

A. "To be completely honest, it is not clear exactly how the medication works."
B. "It increases the level of serotonin in your body, which improves your mood."
C. "It inhibits the reuptake of norepinephrine and serotonin to stabilize mood."
D. "It modifies the amount of dopamine and serotonin your body uses."

57. The nurse is conducting a medication reconciliation for an older adult patient who is prescribed benztropine (Cogentin) for Parkinson disease. Which medication would be contraindicated for this patient?

A. Polyethylene glycol (Miralax)
B. Acetaminophen (Tylenol)
C. Pseudoephedrine (Sudafed)
D. Ondansetron (Zofran)

58. An older adult patient with dementia-related psychosis is prescribed chlorpromazine (Thorazine). The nurse understands that the boxed warning associated with this clinical scenario indicates that the patient is at an increased risk of:

A. Death
B. Worsened dementia
C. Suicidal ideation
D. Stroke

59. The physical therapist is planning to take a patient with Parkinson disease to the hospital gym for some exercise. To facilitate the patient's ability to participate in the activity, the nurse plans to administer the prescribed immediate-release carbidopa/levodopa (Sinemet):

A. One hour prior to the scheduled activity
B. Four hours prior to the scheduled activity
C. Eight hours prior to the scheduled activity
D. The night before the scheduled activity

60. A patient with schizophrenia has been very agitated, and the current medications are not improving the symptoms. The provider orders loxapine (Adasuve). Fifteen minutes after administering the medication to the patient, the nurse returns to evaluate the patient. What is the most important action for the nurse to perform?

A. Administer a second antipsychotic if symptoms persist
B. Perform a complete respiratory assessment
C. Draw a blood specimen to check the drug level
D. Obtain a full set of vital signs and patient weight

61. The nurse is educating the caregiver of an older adult patient regarding the prescribed medication memantine (Namenda). The nurse explains that the medication's dose will increase over the next couple of weeks. How should the nurse describe the expected medication dose schedule to the caregiver?

A. "The dose will be increased weekly until the target dose is met."
B. "The patient will return to the clinic every 4 weeks for a dose increase."
C. "An increased dose will be administered every other day."
D. "The dose will depend on the patient's ability to draw a clock."

62. A patient is admitted to the facility with anxiety and germaphobia (mysophobia). The patient is cooperative and calm at this time, but they do not want to remove their mask due to the fear of contracting an illness from others. Which action should the nurse take?

A. Allow the patient to keep their mask on at all times to ease their anxiety
B. Ask the other patients on the unit to wear masks as well
C. Explain that medical illnesses are rarely present in psychiatric facilities
D. Assign distancing anytime the patient is outside of their room

63. The nurse has completed two sessions with a school-age patient, teaching skills that can be used to redirect inappropriate behaviors. When the nurse observes the patient interacting with other patients, the patient's behavior is unchanged and the new skills are not demonstrated. What intervention should the nurse use first to address the fact that the patient is not using the new skills they were taught?

A. Call the provider and request a pharmaceutical intervention to treat the behaviors
B. Conduct a role-play session with the patient that mimics the observed behavior
C. Restrict the patient's privileges to individual activities within the nurse's sight only
D. Tell the patient that they are extremely unhappy and disappointed in them

64. The nurse and mental health technician are attempting to de-escalate a patient who is extremely agitated, threatening staff, and demonstrating aggressive behavior. The patient is not responding to any of the therapeutic techniques the nurse has attempted. The patient has a history of physical abuse, so the nurse wants to ensure all nonrestrictive measures are exhausted before the patient is physically restrained. What action should the nurse take first?

A. Allow the patient to go to another unit to see if they are more comfortable there
B. Change the current oral antipsychotic medication to intramuscular (IM) and immediately administer
C. Make an announcement asking all available hospital staff to report to the unit
D. Swap the current mental health technician with a different technician who may be less intimidating

65. A pediatric patient with encopresis and chronic constipation presents for a follow-up visit with a parent. The parent reports they are consistently following the treatment plan that was given to them and things are improving. What is the first noninvasive action the nurse should perform to evaluate the status of the condition?

A. Review the monthly stool diary
B. Perform a digital rectal examination
C. Measure abdominal circumference
D. Obtain patient height and weight

66. A patient with a history of post-traumatic stress disorder presents to the mental health facility with family members to assess the patient's progress. The family members report that there has been an improvement in behavior but that the patient's decision-making has drastically declined. The family members inquire about the possibility of a conservatorship. Which of the following is the most appropriate response by the nurse?

A. "Can you describe the current status of the patient's personal matters?"
B. "Has the patient expressed interest in a conservatorship?"
C. "Do you consider the spending habits of the patient to be excessive?"
D. "Have there been any violent outbursts or episodes of self-harm?"

67. A patient was recently diagnosed with bipolar disorder and started on lamotrigine (Lamictal). The patient has an extensive history of hypersexual behavior and high-risk sexual activity. Which of the following would be the best question for the nurse to ask to determine treatment effectiveness?

A. "Have you had more than one sexual partner in the past month?"
B. "How many times have you had sex with your spouse this week?"
C. "Have you had sexually transmitted infection (STI) testing?"
D. "Can you tell me about your sexual encounters recently?"

68. A patient with agoraphobia approaches the nurse to discuss their progress. The patient feels they have improved and would like to start volunteering at a local flower nursery. Which of the following responses by the nurse would best assess the patient's readiness?

A. "Are you sure you feel like you are ready for this type of activity?"
B. "How long has it been since you started cognitive behavioral therapy?"
C. "What made you decide to volunteer at at flower nursery?"
D. "Have you discussed your diagnosis with the supervisor at the flower nursery?"

69. The nurse is working with a patient whose child died of cancer. The patient has had moderate symptoms since the incident despite being compliant with the treatment plan. To evaluate for dysfunctional grieving, the nurse should:

A. Evaluate the patient's relationships with other children
B. Establish when the symptoms initially began
C. Administer a mood disorder screening tool
D. Ask the patient to set goals for the grieving process

70. After completing a psychiatric assessment of a patient, the nurse differentiates bipolar I disorder from bipolar II disorder because:

A. At least one major depressive episode has been documented
B. One past hospitalization for mania has occurred
C. There is a history of suicide attempt
D. There has been one identifiable episode of mania

71. The nurse is completing an initial patient interview. The patient complains of being "down in the dumps" and is pulling and rubbing their skin, has difficulty sitting still, and is wringing their hands. The patient is exhibiting signs of:

A. Comorbid generalized anxiety disorder
B. Compulsions related to obsessive-compulsive disorder
C. Psychomotor agitation
D. Atypical features of major depressive disorder

72. During an initial psychiatric interview, a patient reports that this is their first time being evaluated for possible hospitalization and that they have no past history of psychiatric diagnosis, even after admitting to suicidal ideation. The nurse has determined that the patient has not slept for more than 2 hours at a time, has been told by others that they talk excessively, and has been easily distracted over the past week. Based on this information, the nurse suspects bipolar I disorder over bipolar II disorder because there is:

A. Evidence of mania
B. History of suicide attempt
C. At least one major depressive episode
D. No history of psychiatric inpatient admissions

73. Prior to starting a patient with bipolar disorder with mania on a mood stabilizer, the patient should be evaluated to rule out a thyroid disorder based on the patient's symptoms, which include tremor, tachycardia, profuse sweating, and:

A. Weight gain
B. Abdominal pain
C. Dry mouth
D. Weight loss

74. Prior to starting a patient on an antidepressant for major depressive disorder, the patient should be evaluated to rule out a thyroid disorder based on the patient's symptoms, which include low mood, lethargy, weight gain, and:

A. Tachycardia
B. Cold intolerance
C. Difficulty sleeping
D. Pruritis

75. The nurse is assessing a 6-year-old patient who is cognitively impaired, makes poor eye contact, and does not interact socially with peers. The patient's mother took medications for a seizure disorder and depression while pregnant. To determine exposure to a neurologic teratogen, the nurse will assess for:

A. Spina bifida at birth
B. History of cleft palate
C. Congenital Ebstein anomaly
D. Neonatal withdrawal syndrome

76. The nurse is working in the psychiatric emergency department when a patient with a history of bipolar disorder who takes valproate (Depakote) comes in with a red maculopapular rash. The patient reports being started on a new medication. The medication the nurse suspects to be the cause for these symptoms is:

A. Lithium carbonate (Lithobid)
B. Lurasidone (Latuda)
C. Cariprazine (Vraylar)
D. Lamotrigine (Lamictal)

77. A patient diagnosed with bipolar disorder is taking carbamazepine (Tegretol). The patient suddenly develops a fever, sore throat, and oral ulcerations. The patient's white blood cell count is 2,800 mm^3, and the absolute neutrophil count is 1,400 mm^3. The nurse understands that the patient is currently experiencing:
   A. Neuroleptic malignant syndrome
   B. Serotonin syndrome
   C. Agranulocytosis
   D. Carbamazepine overdose

78. A patient presenting to the emergency department with chest pain and prolonged QRS waves on EKG has a reported history of taking "something for depression." The patient denies using any other medications. With no history of substance use, the nurse suspects that the antidepressant the patient uses is:
   A. Escitalopram (Lexapro)
   B. Vilazodone (Viibryd)
   C. Trazodone (Desyrel)
   D. Imipramine (Tofranil)

79. A patient taking a selective serotonin reuptake inhibitor (SSRI) reports daytime somnolence that is affecting their job. The best action to take at this time is to:
   A. Schedule an appointment to have the dose or medication changed
   B. Adjust the time of the administration of the SSRI
   C. Discuss mild to moderate use of caffeine during the day
   D. Suggest adding melatonin at night to improve sleep

80. The nurse is practicing within ethical standards of practice and protecting patient rights when:
   A. Disclosing the medical diagnosis to the patient's adult child
   B. Checking a hospitalized friend's medical records for test results
   C. Sending a deceased patient's medical records to an attorney upon request
   D. Participating in interprofessional meetings about treatment

81. The nurse demonstrates a clear understanding of the ethical scope and standard of practice by:

    A. Participating on a hospital committee to ensure that patients with substance use disorders have equal access to care
    B. Informing a voluntarily hospitalized patient that they do not have the right to request to be discharged against medical advice
    C. Deciding not to notify someone whom a patient has stated they wish to harm because the potential victim lives out of state
    D. Failing to report illegal actions taken toward a patient in a mental health clinic because of fear of retribution

82. The psychiatric–mental health nurse is reviewing the treatment plan of an adolescent patient who was just diagnosed with major depressive disorder and placed on an antidepressant. When providing patient education, the nurse would begin with the most important information, which is that the medication:

    A. Will take 4 to 6 weeks to take effect
    B. Will be started at a low dose due to the patient's age
    C. Carries a risk of serotonin syndrome
    D. May cause activation of suicidal thoughts

83. The nurse is assessing a patient who reports difficulty initiating and maintaining sleep 4 to 5 days per week, which affects the patient's ability to perform well at work. The nurse should educate the patient regarding:

    A. Sleep hygiene
    B. Mood record
    C. PHQ-9
    D. GAD-7 screening tool

84. A patient has just been prescribed phenelzine (Nardil) for treatment-resistant depression. To help the patient avoid a potentially life-threatening adverse effect, the nurse includes in the medication education that:

    A. A slow titration schedule for the medication is necessary
    B. The patient should take the medication at night to avoid sedation and prevent falls
    C. The medication must be tapered gradually when discontinuing
    D. The patient should avoid consuming foods that are high in tyramine

85. The nurse is educating a patient regarding lithium toxicity. The nurse concludes that the patient has understood the education when the patient states that they will report:

A. Persistent nausea and vomiting
B. Constant diarrhea
C. Hyperthermia
D. Uncontrolled shivering

86. The nurse is educating a patient regarding monoamine oxidase inhibitors (MAOIs), including that concurrent consumption of tyramine-containing foods will induce a hypertensive crisis. The nurse realizes that the education was effective when the patient reports that they will not consume:

A. Ripe bananas
B. Smoked salmon
C. Vodka tonic
D. Chicken breast

87. The disorder consistent with a patient's decreased free thyroxine (T4) and elevated thyroid-stimulating hormone (TSH) level is:

A. Primary hypothyroidism
B. Hyperthyroidism
C. Acute thyroiditis
D. Secondary hypothyroidism

88. When monitoring a patient on lithium, the laboratory value that would warrant immediate attention is:

A. Glomerular filtration rate of 90
B. Serum creatinine of 2.0 mg/dL
C. Free thyroxine of 0.8 ng/dL
D. Thyroid-stimulating hormone of 5.0 mU/L

89. For the psychiatric–mental health nurse to diagnose a patient with generalized anxiety disorder (GAD), the patient must have experienced the symptoms of GAD for at least:

A. 3 months
B. 2 weeks
C. 6 months
D. 1 year

90. To be considered for diagnosis, major depressive symptoms must be present for at least:

A. 1 year
B. 2 weeks
C. 6 months
D. 3 months

91. An older adult patient presents with chronic confusion and depressed mood. The patient's spouse reports that the patient has a history of excessive drinking as a younger adult. To determine whether the symptoms stem from Alzheimer dementia or a common chronic condition associated with alcohol use, the most appropriate laboratory test would be:

A. Complete blood count
B. Thiamine level
C. Basic metabolic panel
D. Folic acid level

92. To help differentiate between bipolar I and bipolar II disorders, the nurse asks a patient who presents with rapid speech, distractibility, and decreased need for sleep:

A. "Do you feel you are unstoppable?"
B. "How long do your symptoms last?"
C. "Are you easily distracted?"
D. "Do you feel depressed?"

93. To help differentiate bipolar disorder from attention deficit hyperactivity disorder (ADHD), the nurse asks:

A. "Do your symptoms occur episodically?"
B. "Are you easily distracted?"
C. "Do your friends say you talk too fast?"
D. "Would you say your symptoms are troubling?"

94. A patient presents with being easily distracted, having rapid speech, and expressing a flight of ideas. The patient states, "The voices tell me I am God." The patient's friend reports that prior to this, the patient was severely depressed for months with feelings of guilt, worthlessness, and hypersomnia, but now the patient can't seem to sleep and has been up for 4 days straight. The nurse suspects a diagnosis of:

A. Major depressive disorder
B. Bipolar I disorder
C. Bipolar II disorder
D. Brief psychotic episode

95. A young adult patient was discharged from a drug and alcohol program after spending 12 weeks detoxing from alcohol and opioids. After discharge, the patient understood the need to make lifestyle changes to continue supporting progress. An example of a healthy change the patient can make to support recovery is to:

A. Return to employment at the local distillery
B. Spend time at home reflecting on what was learned in recovery
C. Enroll in a psychology course at the local community college
D. Apply for a position as a receptionist at the pain clinic near home

96. When meeting a patient suffering from trauma for the first time, the nurse would first:

A. Introduce themself and provide background
B. Briefly discuss the therapeutic process
C. Ensure that the patient feels safe and secure
D. Obtain history and discuss treatment options

97. An older adult patient presents for an initial intake for depression. During the history-taking process, the patient admits to previously being in rehab for alcohol use disorder and having relapsed several times. The screening tool to administer to assess the patient for alcoholism is the:

A. CAGE questionnaire
B. CIWA scale
C. Hamilton Scale for Depression
D. *DSM-5* to assess the criteria for alcoholism

98. A screening questionnaire used to identify adverse incidents that occurred during a patient's childhood and that increase the patient's likelihood to suffer lifelong consequences is:

A. ACE
B. MMSE
C. CAI
D. YMRS

99. An older adult patient presents in order to address depression and anxiety symptoms that have been getting progressively worse after a myocardial infarction 3 months ago. The medication that is contraindicated for this patient is:

A. Amitriptyline (Elavil)
B. Sertraline (Zoloft)
C. Fluoxetine (Prozac)
D. Lamotrigine (Lamictal)

100. The "G" in the CAGE questionnaire indicates:

A. Gluttony
B. Guilt
C. Greed
D. Gauge

101. A patient reports being 3 months sober from opioids. A toxicology screening is indicated upon noting that the patient:

A. Appears tired but is easily arousable
B. Has pinpoint pupils
C. Appears disheveled
D. Reports feeling constipated

102. When using the CAGE questionnaire, the nurse will ask the patient:

A. "Do you enjoy drinking?"
B. "Do you ever feel you should cut down on your drinking?"
C. "What made you decide to cut down on your drinking?"
D. "Do you think you have a drinking problem?"

103. An older adult patient comes into the office for an initial visit. After assessment and evaluation, the patient is given a diagnosis of major depressive disorder, and prescription medication is recommended. The patient explains that it is "against my religion" to take any medications for this condition. In an effort to promote cultural competence, the nurse:

A. Advises the patient that they must take the medication in order to feel better
B. Has a member of another religious group discuss the treatment plan with the patient
C. Documents this as refusal of treatment and discusses the implications of refusing
D. Spends more time discussing the patient's religion and how it may impact decision-making

104. After working with a family with significantly dysfunctional patterns, the nurse observes that the teenage daughter begins to show signs of self-differentiation. This would be observed by the patient:

A. Continuing to feel enmeshed in family boundaries
B. Feeling she has self-worth despite her family relationships
C. Feeling that she has continued low self-worth
D. Showing that she is developing self-identity

105. An older adult patient presents to the office for treatment. The nurse demonstrates their role in patient advocacy by:

A. Ensuring that the patient has a trusted family member with whom to discuss the treatment plan
B. Discussing the treatment plan with the patient's family without the patient's consent
C. Disregarding information regarding the patient's healthcare power of attorney
D. Prescribing medications without allowing time for the patient to ask questions

106. The family system has reached homeostasis when the family:

A. Continues with maladaptive communication
B. Returns to stability despite continuing dysfunction
C. Continues with the same behaviors as previously
D. Communicates less effectively among its members

107. The key concepts of structural family therapy are:

A. Reframing and paradoxical interventions
B. Family structure, subsystems, and boundaries
C. Homeostasis and feedback loops
D. Emotions and attachment styles

108. Self-differentiation, which is an important concept in family systems theory, means the:

A. Level achieved when one's self-worth is not dependent on external relationships
B. Ability to differentiate problematic traits among family members
C. Relabeling of problematic self-fulfilling behaviors to have more positive meaning
D. Attempt to break contact between self and family members

109. An older adult patient begins to recognize patterns of familial dysfunction with poor communication and convinces their family to commit to family therapy. Interventions with an approach in strategic family therapy focus on:

A. Family structure to effectively manage problems
B. The problem and the sequence of interactions that maintain the problem
C. Self-confrontation of each family member
D. Self-differentiation of each family member

110. The stages of the transtheoretical model of change include:

A. Contemplation, freezing, unfreezing, and action
B. Precontemplation, contemplation, preparation, action, and maintenance
C. Plan, do, study, act, and maintain
D. Freezing, transition, action, unfreezing, and maintenance

111. The psychiatric–mental health nurse has a follow-up visit with a teenage patient. Upon evaluation, the patient states that they were using marijuana occasionally to cope with anxiety but now use it daily to get through the day. The nurse understands that the patient is still in the precontemplation phase of change when the patient:

A. Plans to stop using marijuana next month
B. States that their marijuana use is not a big deal
C. Agrees to reduce marijuana use before the next visit
D. States that the marijuana use is a problem but they do not know how to stop

112. The nurse sees a patient for an initial visit with concern for alcohol use disorder. The statement that identifies that the patient is in the contemplation stage of change is:

A. "My drinking is not a problem for me at all. That's not the reason why I am here today."
B. "My drinking is a problem, and I'm thinking about how to improve in the next few months."
C. "My drinking has always been a problem, but I'm not sure if it can get better at this point."
D. "My alcohol use is not something that I need any help with at this time."

113. In general, the neurotransmitter dopamine is increased in patients with:

A. Parkinson disease
B. Depression
C. Schizophrenia
D. Attention deficit hyperactivity disorder

114. The suprachiasmatic nucleus is located in the:

A. Amygdala
B. Pineal gland
C. Hypothalamus
D. Hippocampus

115. According to the *DSM-5*, diagnostic criteria for major depressive disorder (MDD) include:

A. Three symptoms of depression for the same 2-week period
B. Fatigue or loss of energy nearly every day for 2 weeks
C. Marked disinterest in activities for most of the day, every day for 1 week
D. Restlessness or feeling on edge for 2 weeks

116. When monitoring a patient taking valproate (Depakote) for treatment of mania in bipolar disorder, the target serum level is between:

A. 350 and 450 ng/mL
B. 50 and 125 mcg/mL
C. 0.8 and 1.2 mEq/L
D. 0.1 and 1.5 mEq/L

117. When treating a patient with antipsychotics, it is important for the nurse to know that the peak plasma concentration after an oral dose is reached in how many hours?

A. 1 to 2
B. 2 to 3
C. 6 to 8
D. 12 to 16

118. Self-liberation is a process found in the behavioral change stage of:

A. Precontemplation
B. Contemplation
C. Preparation
D. Action

119. After receiving the order to discharge a patient, the nurse meets with the patient to review the discharge plan and provide education on the discharge medications. Initially, the patient demonstrates interest in receiving the information. As the nurse continues to review the information, the patient does not appear to be paying attention. The patient begins to avoid eye contact, does not have any questions, and does not review the discharge instructions or the literature. The most likely reason for the changes in the patient's behavior is that the:

A. Patient cannot read and needs pictures
B. Patient does not want to be discharged
C. Materials are not written at the correct grade level
D. Patient is responding to internal stimuli

120. The provider discontinues venlafaxine (Effexor) because of lack of positive response from the patient. The nurse advises the patient to expect the possibility of symptoms such as nausea, dizziness, "shock-like feeling," irritability, tremor, confusion, headache, or sweating. The nurse is reviewing symptoms of:

A. Discontinuation syndrome
B. Influenza
C. Panic attack
D. Sleep deprivation

121. At 8:00 p.m., the nurse evaluates a patient who has been using heroin and morphine for over a year. The patient reports that last use was "around lunchtime." The nurse can anticipate that the patient may exhibit early signs of physical withdrawal, such as:

A. Increased lacrimation, rhinorrhea, and piloerection
B. Pinpoint pupils and bradycardia
C. Tonic-clonic seizures and tremors
D. Dysthymia, vivid, unpleasant dreams, and insomnia

122. A teenage patient expresses confidence in their ability to avoid smoking and to exercise regularly to prevent pulmonary disease. This statement is an example of:

A. Self-efficacy
B. Unrealistic optimism
C. Self-liberation
D. Dramatic relief

123. An older adult has recently developed negative feelings toward his son. The father thinks that the son is avoiding him and not caring for him properly. This is a recent thought pattern for the father, and he has not experienced any previous mental disturbance. The son brings the father to the mental health facility to seek help to improve their relationship. The nurse finds that the father's feelings and expectations have developed because of excessive movie watching. The therapy that can be used for this patient is:

A. Humanistic
B. Cognitive behavioral
C. Interpersonal
D. Psychodynamic

124. A nonprofit organization is planning an initiative to assist older adults in leading a more healthy and active lifestyle. The initiative will last 6 months and includes monthly counseling sessions, seminars, and collaboration with a top healthcare facility. The planned long-term outcome of this project is to:

A. Collaborate with a well-regarded hospital
B. Assess the number of patients treated
C. Help patients achieve a healthier lifestyle
D. Create detailed literature about the project

125. A child with academic issues is brought to the mental health facility. The child does not want to study mathematics because they scored low on previous tests. The child is also not interested in attending their guitar and drawing lessons. The crisis that must resolve for the advancement of the child is:

A. Trust versus mistrust
B. Autonomy versus shame and doubt
C. Initiation versus guilt
D. Industry versus inferiority

126. An adult patient is brought to the emergency department (ED) for erratic behavior. Previous ED history includes serious headaches, fatigue, and transient blurry vision 3 months ago. Recently, the patient was prescribed 40 to 60 mg per day of prednisone for approximately 1 month; then the dose was tapered. Anxiety and poor sleep were reported during that time, and depressive episode was denied. The patient has not slept for more than 3 hours a night for over a week. Mood is irritable, with no cognitive deficits. Although affect is labile, it is appropriate to the content of the patient's speech (e.g., the patient becomes tearful when reporting pending divorce). Speech is loud, pressured, and overelaborative. No perceptual disturbances are reported or observed. Exhibited mental status examination abnormalities include flight of ideas, racing thoughts, increased energy, and being easily distractible. The patient is oriented to time and place and convincingly denies suicidal and homicidal ideation. The patient exhibits poor judgment, and insight is absent. Based on medical and psychiatric history and current mental status findings, the nurse suspects:

A. Adjustment disorder with mixed anxiety and depressed mood
B. Bipolar II
C. Bipolar I
D. Steroid psychosis

127. A patient reports feeling depressed due to stress at work and describes how the stress causes body aches and general malaise. The nurse asks the patient to monitor and record heart rate and blood pressure when experiencing stress. The patient is also instructed to perform certain stretching exercises to reduce the muscle tension. This type of behavior therapy is called:

A. Exposure
B. Aversion
C. Biofeedback
D. Modeling

128. A patient with a fear of dogs comes to the clinic and reports increasing obsession about the phobia. The patient has started to feel extremely anxious whenever leaving home. A possible therapy treatment option for this patient would be:

A. Psychoanalytical
B. Exposure
C. Dream analysis
D. Aversion

129. A child enrolled in a dance class is unable to learn the steps. One day, the child trips, becomes very self-conscious, and has still more difficulty learning the steps. Eventually the child stops attending the class. The probable unresolved crisis is:

A. Integrity versus despair
B. Autonomy versus shame and doubt
C. Trust versus mistrust
D. Intimacy versus isolation

130. The first-line treatment for attention deficit hyperactivity disorder (ADHD) includes:

A. Psychostimulants
B. Second-generation antipsychotics
C. First-generation antipsychotics
D. Anticonvulsants

131. The cholinesterase inhibitor used to treat both Alzheimer disease and Parkinson disease is:

A. Donepezil
B. Rivastigmine
C. Galantamine
D. Paraoxon

132. The potential long-term adverse effects of lithium treatment include:

A. Hypothyroidism
B. Thrombocytopenia
C. Hepatic failure
D. Pancreatitis

133. A patient with bipolar disorder has been prescribed lithium and several other medications. The nurse educates the patient about lithium toxicity to help with self-assessment. The nurse mentions symptoms such as:

A. Weight loss
B. High blood pressure
C. Insomnia
D. Blurred vision

134. The monoamine oxidase inhibitor (MAOI) found as a transdermal patch is:

A. Phenelzine (Nardil)
B. Selegiline (Eldepryl)
C. Isocarboxazid (Marplan)
D. Tranylcypromine (Parnate)

135. Ramelteon (Rozerem) is often prescribed to treat:

A. Sleep paralysis
B. Anxiety
C. Insomnia
D. Paranoia

136. Typical antipsychotics help in alleviating:

A. Delusions and hallucinations in schizophrenia
B. Mixed episodes of bipolar disorder
C. Manic episodes of bipolar disorder
D. Difficulty staying asleep in insomnia

137. The antidepressant drug used to treat insomnia is:

A. Bupropion (Wellbutrin)
B. Mirtazapine (Remeron)
C. Fluoxetine (Prozac)
D. Duloxetine (Cymbalta)

138. The antidepressant drug paroxetine (Paxil) belongs to the group of:

A. Benzodiazepines
B. Beta-blockers
C. Serotonin and norepinephrine reuptake inhibitors
D. Selective serotonin reuptake inhibitors

139. The drug that acts as a norepinephrine and serotonin-specific antidepressant is:

A. Paroxetine (Paxil)
B. Mirtazapine (Remeron)
C. Bupropion (Wellbutrin)
D. Vortioxetine (Trintellix)

140. The single element that is widely regarded as the gold standard among mood stabilizers used to treat patients with bipolar disorder is:

A. Sodium
B. Potassium
C. Lithium
D. Monoamine oxidase

141. Chlorpromazine (Thorazine) was the first pharmacotherapeutic:

A. Antipsychotic
B. Analgesic
C. Antipyretic
D. Antispasmodic

142. The type of medication used for Alzheimer disease is:

A. Muscle blockers
B. Cholinesterase inhibitors
C. Antipsychotics
D. Lithium

143. Pharmacokinetics is the study of the:

A. Effect of a medication on the body
B. Absorption, distribution, transformation, and removal of a drug from the body
C. Influence of genetic factors on a person's response to medications
D. Prevention of the adverse effects of various medications

144. Atomoxetine (Straterra) is used to treat children with:

A. Attention deficit hyperactivity disorder
B. Schizophrenia
C. Depression
D. Bipolar disorder

145. A patient with bipolar disorder visits the clinic and reports severe stress along with anger issues. There has been a decline in appetite, sleep, and energy level of the patient since the last visit. Along with medications, the type of therapy that would be beneficial for this patient would be:

A. Family
B. Behavioral
C. Cognitive behavioral
D. Interpersonal

146. Alprazolam (Xanax) is a benzodiazepine that functions by enhancing the effects of:

A. Serotonin
B. Dopamine
C. Gamma-aminobutyric acid (GABA)
D. Melatonin

147. A patient comes to the office for the first time and wants advice about family problems. The patient states that the problems are affecting their work life and suddenly begins crying. The nurse should:

A. Ask the patient to stop crying and then place a box of tissues near the patient
B. Let the patient cry for some time and then discuss the issues after the patient settles
C. Ask the patient to go outside to cry for some time and then return
D. Let the patient cry and then comfort the patient with a hug after some time

148. A patient with problems in their marriage visits the mental health facility. The patient tells the nurse that they have had conflicts in their marriage before, but they used to figure out the solutions themselves. However, this time, the spouse of the patient has started bringing their best friend into every fight to direct any communication toward the patient. The patient explains that they feel uncomfortable due to the spouse's friend's interventions. This situation is an example of:

A. Triangulation
B. Modeling
C. Cross-generational coalition
D. Covert coalition

149. An adult patient who has been treated with lithium for bipolar disorder for more than 3 years reports feeling weak and experiencing cold intolerance, constipation, and weight gain during the past 6 months. Physical examination shows dry, coarse skin and bradycardia, hypothermia, and swelling of the hands and feet. The diagnostic study the nurse anticipates is:

A. Blood alcohol level

B. Serum thyroid-stimulating hormone

C. Liver function testing

D. EKG

150. An adult patient with a history of bipolar disorder and type 2 diabetes reports a 25-lb weight gain, especially in the abdominal area. Their HbA1C is 10.6%, and the lipid profile indicates total cholesterol of 240 mg/dL and low-density lipoprotein of 200 mg/dL. The patient reports that they started a new medication 6 months ago. The most likely medication is:

A. Citalopram (Celexa)

B. Olanzapine (Zyprexa)

C. Dextroamphetamine (Adderall)

D. Sertraline (Zoloft)

Practice Examination Answers With Rationales

1. A) Join family dinners even if just to sit at the dinner table

The patient joining the family at dinnertime will give the family a chance to sit together and share thoughts. If the patient stops engaging in family activities when sad, it may create a distance between the patient and other family members. The discontinuation or alteration of the medication regimen is done only after an evaluation by the prescribing provider, and feeling better is not a criterion to discontinue the medication. Sharing feelings is a positive approach that helps the patient connect and realize that they are not alone.

2. C) Interpersonal

Interpersonal therapy improves the interpersonal relationships and social interactions of the patient. Aversion therapy is used to treat issues such as alcohol use disorder, shoplifting, or self-harm. Behavioral therapy changes maladaptive behaviors by targeting problems like gambling, anger issues, or alcohol use disorder. It is also used for disorders like phobias or anxiety. Psychoanalytic therapy assumes that the root cause of mental illness is childhood trauma; it is not considered a valid approach today.

3. D) Biofeedback

The patient measuring vital signs is a part of biofeedback therapy. In this therapy, interventions help in gaining a better understanding of the physiology of the patient, based on which further pharmacological and psychological interventions can be made. Aversion therapy is used when the patient needs to quit a habit like smoking or alcohol misuse. Interpersonal therapy focuses on improving social and personal life by resolving interpersonal conflicts. Modeling therapy focuses on changing the patient's behavior by providing a model to the patient that the patient can then imitate to change concerning behavior.

4. D) Meditation

Meditation is a popular complementary and alternative treatment. Meditation is defined as the intentional self-regulation of attention from moment to moment. This technique calls for an intentional and self-regulated focusing of attention to relax and calm the mind and body. Systematic desensitization/exposure is a form of psychotherapy used for patients with phobias, not generalized anxiety. Electroconvulsive therapy and transcranial magnetic stimulation are medical treatments for treatment-resistant and severe depression.

5. C) Ginkgo biloba

Ginkgo biloba has been used to treat impaired cognition with convincing results, improving cognitive function, neuropsychiatric symptoms associated with age-related cognitive decline, mild cognitive impairment, and mild to moderate dementia. Valerian (*Valeriana officinalis*) treats anxiety and insomnia. Melatonin is used for the regulation of sleep. Intake of omega-3 fatty acids is thought to lower the risk of developing major depression, prenatal depression, and bipolar depression.

6. D) Suicidal behavior

Suicide is the leading cause of death in schizophrenic patients. A command hallucination is a false perception of instructions or orders the patient may feel obligated to obey or unable to resist. The content of the command auditory hallucinations may include messages to self-harm. Command hallucinations and persecutory hallucinations are associated with a high risk for suicidal behavior. The assessment of the risk for self-harm is the priority. Monitoring medication compliance is important because nonadherence may be contributing to the current mental state, but it is not the main priority. Aripiprazole is a second-generation atypical psychotic with well-documented risks for metabolic syndrome. Monitoring for all side effects is an important component of care to assess the overall health of the patient, but it does not present an imminent risk for loss of life. Refocusing the patient on reality is a therapeutic intervention and should be included in the plan of care. However, the priority is the suicidal assessment.

7. A) Autonomy

Autonomy is the ethical principle in which people respect the rights of others to make their own decisions. The patient has the right to decide whether to continue the pregnancy, so the situation falls under the autonomy principle. Beneficence can be defined as the duty to benefit or promote the health and well-being of others. The quality of being honest or truthful is veracity. Fidelity involves commitment and loyalty to a patient.

8. A) Beneficence

The nurse helping the patient feel calm before administering the drug shows beneficence. It is promoting the good of the patient. The nurse must administer the drug but also act to benefit the patient. Justice involves providing an equitable distribution of resources or care without prejudice or differentiation. Autonomy allows the patient to refuse a treatment or to prefer a certain treatment plan. The patient is not refusing the drug or requesting a different one. Veracity is the truthful communication of relevant information related to the drug or treatment to the patient.

9. B) Drug-induced liver injury

The patient's symptoms are acute, not chronic. Medications such as valproic acid (Depakote) are common causes of acute liver injury. Some forms of gallbladder disease, such as choledocholithiasis (a stone in the bile duct), present acutely with jaundice, fever, and loss of appetite, but they are associated with severe abdominal pain. The acute presentation is not consistent with primary biliary cirrhosis, a chronic liver disease usually occurring in the 40- to 50-year-old age-group. The clinical picture, particularly the lab results, do not suggest a blood dyscrasia.

10. A) Self-awareness

The nurse understands that values and beliefs guide behavior, but self-awareness helps them to accept the uniqueness and differences among beliefs. Self-awareness is self-knowledge—knowledge about one's own actions. Values are abstract standards and represent an ideal, either positive or negative. A belief is a concept that is held as true by a person. It is not the rational concept of believing in something to be true. Supervision is an important factor in building ethically and legally sound therapeutic relationships. Supervision involves a third person supervising or looking over the behavior of the nurse. In this case, the relationship is between the nurse and the patient only.

11. B) Clonidine

Clonidine is an antihypertensive agent and acts as a nonstimulant for ADHD. It acts centrally on the alpha 2 receptors found in the prefrontal cortex. It is also used to treat Tourette syndrome. Amphetamine (D) and methylphenidate (D,L) are recommended to patients with ADHD; however, these drugs should be avoided if the patient is also diagnosed with Tourette syndrome because they may worsen that condition. Diazepam is a sedating medication that is not a primary treatment of Tourette syndrome.

12. A) Armodafinil

Armodafinil, a wakefulness-promoting drug, would be used to treat this patient. It functions by boosting hypothalamic wakefulness center activity. Clomipramine, desipramine, and diazepam are sleep-inducing drugs beneficial in treating insomnia and therefore are not recommended for excessive drowsiness.

13. B) Was experiencing extrapyramidal symptoms

The patient has experienced extrapyramidal symptoms due to use of an antipsychotic drug. This usually occurs young adults and is treated with anticholinergic drugs to increase the transmission of dopamine blocked by the antipsychotic. An overdose of antipsychotics causes an altered state of consciousness, excess salivation, and respiratory depression. Myocarditis should be suspected only if troponin levels are elevated and other related features are observed. Clozapine should be stopped in cases such as when C-reactive protein level is higher than 100 mg/L.

14. B) Carbamazepine

Stevens–Johnson syndrome is a life-threatening side effect of carbamazepine, which is recommended for bipolar disorder. Headache, insomnia, and anxiety are adverse effects of armodafinil, which is prescribed for wakefulness promotion. Hepatic dysfunction, renal dysfunction, and blood dyscrasias are rare but life-threatening side effects of chlordiazepoxide, which is prescribed for alcohol withdrawal symptoms. Dry mouth, dizziness, major depression, and sedation are side effects of clonidine, which is prescribed for hypertension.

15. D) Blocking the reuptake of serotonin

Selective serotonin reuptake inhibitors (SSRIs) block the reuptake of serotonin by blocking the 5-HT2 receptors. Blocking the reuptake of these neurotransmitters makes them available at the synapse in a larger quantity, which helps in alleviating depression. Stimulating the effects of GABA inhibits neuronal activity and is used to treat seizure disorders. Reuptake of norepinephrine and dopamine would not help because their presence at the synapse is needed to alleviate depression.

16. C) Lithium (Lithobid)

Lithium is approved by U.S. Food and Drug Administration (FDA) for treating acute mania. Lithium has incredible clinical benefits but can be highly toxic due to the small therapeutic window. The second-generation antipsychotic drug lurasidone is used for treating bipolar depression and is known to be less toxic. Cariprazine is an FDA-approved drug that does not fall into the most toxic category. Lamotrigine is an antipsychotic drug recommended for treating bipolar depression that has fewer side effects than lithium and is generally safe.

17. C) Is not harmful to themself or others

There are exceptional cases in which the nurse can share information revealed during a session with someone outside of the session. When the patient does not show any sign of harm to self or others, the nurse should maintain confidentiality. However, when the patient is suicidal and may cause self-harm, for protection of the patient, the nurse should connect with concerned persons or authorities. When the nurse notices abuse such as domestic violence or child abuse, the nurse must report that to a third party. When the nurse learns that the patient may harm a known person, the nurse should inform that person and other concerned authorities.

18. B) Switch their phones off completely during the session

Technology usage can be a challenge to confidentiality in group therapy. To avoid leakage of the information shared by members of the group, phones should be put in switched-off mode. Putting the phones on silent mode does not ensure confidentiality because the phones can still be used to take photos or record audio. Group members often share conversations beyond sessions; there is no reason to forbid this. Asking the members to not talk with each other outside the group can affect the purpose of the therapy.

19. C) Patients who feel autonomous and independent are more receptive to treatment and have more successful outcomes

Autonomy and independence are integral components of self-determination, and patients who feel empowered by these characteristics will be more receptive to treatment and thus will have more successful outcomes. While self-determination allows patients to competently make decisions based on understanding their rights, the decision-making is based on competence. Likewise, promoting self-determination is an ethically sound practice; however, irrational decision-making is not always the result, and patients can often make rational, sound decisions. Patients feel more empowered when they feel their rights are being protected and supported, but self-determination is not related only to patient rights.

20. B) Attempt to de-escalate the situation by removing stimulation

The first step the nurse will take is to de-escalate the situation by removing stimuli, talking to the patient calmly and actively listening, and providing a diversion. Administering medication such as diazepam (Valium) would be a possible next step if these interventions are not successful. Referral to a psychiatrist may be needed, but all other attempts should be made to de-escalate the situation first. Asking the family for permission to restrain the patient is not needed legally but would be implemented if the patient is found to cause harm to self or others.

21. C) Cyclothymic

Having a sibling with bipolar I disorder is a risk factor for cyclothymic disorder, a rare type of mood disorder. The risk factor of schizotypal personality disorder is having a relative with schizophrenia. Patients with narcissistic personality disorder generally have relatives with the same disorder. The risk factors for developing conduct disorder involve being rejected or neglected by parents, living in a large family, and consuming alcohol or other substances at home.

22. C) Ask the patient's permission to allow the two people to stay in the room

In order to maintain the confidentiality of the patient, the nurse should seek the patient's permission to allow the two people to stay. If the patient grants permission, the nurse should ask the visitors their names and what relationships they have with the patient before beginning any discussion with the patient. The nurse should not ask the visitors to leave the room before seeking the patient's permission.

23. C) Agoraphobia

The tendency to avoid staying in an enclosed place or standing in line for fear of being trapped is a diagnostic feature of agoraphobia. This disorder also makes one feel panicked in an adverse situation. In major depressive disorder, patients may avoid public transport or leaving the home because they feel a loss of energy and low self-esteem, but fear is not the reason for these behaviors. Kleptomania is an uncontrollable urge to steal. It brings tension before committing the theft but does not bring panic. Feeling challenged to throw away possessions even if they do not have value is a sign of hoarding disorder; it is not related to panic.

24. C) Grandiose

When a patient believes that they possess exceptional abilities that are false or unbelievable, those beliefs are regarded as diagnostic features of grandiose delusion. Erotomanic delusion deals with a false belief of the patient that a person loves the patient romantically. Nihilistic delusion is a reasonless belief that some major catastrophe is about to take place. In persecutory delusion, a patient thinks that other people are trying to harass or harm the patient.

25. D) Ask sensitive questions only when the patient is alone
The family member of a patient can stay with the patient while interviewing, but the nurse should ask sensitive questions only when the patient is alone. The initial action by the nurse should be to establish rapport, not address the fear of dying. The nurse should never address any patient by their first name unless asked to do so by the patient. The nurse should ask if the patient wants to allow their son to stay during the interview and act accordingly.

26. D) Express that it is difficult to understand the feelings of the patient at present
In cases where a patient is experiencing a complex or persistent feeling of grief even after therapies, it is important to acknowledge that the feeling of loss or grief must have been devastating and that it is very difficult for the nurse to understand what the patient must be currently feeling. Sharing a story about a loss in the nurse's own family is not helpful and may be seen as minimizing the patient's feelings. Telling a patient that their child is with God assumes the patient is religious and does not facilitate the grief process. The length of the grief process varies, so the focus should be on addressing the current symptoms as opposed to looking at a suggested timeline.

27. A) Bipolar II
The diagnostic criteria for bipolar II disorder include at least one hypomanic episode and at least one major depressive episode. Therefore, the nurse suspects bipolar II disorder. The diagnostic criteria for bipolar I disorder include these episodes along with one or more manic episodes. Panic disorder is a subset of anxiety disorder. Its diagnostic criteria involve palpitations, dizziness, chest pain, choking, and fear of dying. The criteria for cyclothymic disorder include hypomanic episodes and major depressive episodes, but these do not abide by the diagnostic criteria of major depressive episodes.

28. A) Disruptive mood dysregulation
The diagnostic criteria for disruptive mood dysregulation disorder involve a problem in dealing with anger management. The anger is expressed verbally or physically. The duration of the condition should be 12 months or more. In persistent depressive disorder, the patient experiences symptoms of chronic depression for 2 years or more. People with oppositional defiant disorder often indulge in arguments with others and are easily agitated, frequently blaming their mistakes on other people. The duration for diagnosis of this condition should be at least 6 months. People with intermittent explosive disorder find difficulty in controlling their anger, leading to property destruction or physical assault. The diagnosis for this disorder is made if the patient experiences at least three anger outbursts resulting in harm or destruction over a duration of 12 months.

29. A) Panic
Trembling, sweating, and increased heart rate are some of the diagnostic criteria of panic disorder. The diagnostic criteria of bipolar disorder include hypomanic, manic, and major depressive episodes. Patients with hoarding disorder face difficulty in parting from their possessions and fear the distress that parting with them may induce. Excoriation disorder includes diagnostic criteria such as the presence of skin lesions and repeated acts of skin picking.

30. D) Patient's problem-solving skills have deteriorated
Deterioration of problem-solving skills is associated with impaired coping. Social isolation causes feelings of being rejected and not being good enough. Spiritual distress makes one angry toward a greater power, and impaired sexual functioning can change sexual patterns. To determine the condition of impaired coping in a patient, the nurse should question the problem-solving skills of the patient.

31. A) Grant each other's requests only after keeping some strings attached
Granting a request while keeping strings attached is a type of manipulation. An example of distraction is talking about irrelevant things when family problems are being discussed. Accusing each other is known as blaming, not manipulating. Acting well-meaning in front of other family members is an example of placating.

32. C) Express that they are sorry for the loss and show interest in knowing more
The nurse should take an empathetic approach when a patient describes a loss. Responses that involve feeling sorry about the loss and showing interest in knowing more about the situation express empathy and help the patient to clarify their feelings. In certain cases, the loss of a parent or family member may not be upsetting; in fact, it might be a relief for the patient, so it is preferable not to state that the loss is upsetting when asking the patient to share further. Rather than asking specifically about the patient's feelings, the nurse should ask about the whole situation or story as a means to better understand the patient's feelings. The nurse's approach should be empathetic first, and after the end of the interview, the patient may be given reassurance as appropriate.

33. D) Has developed a feeling of isolation
Feeling of isolation is related to hopelessness. The problem of impaired coping brings issues in problem-solving and can cause a person to develop addiction issues with drugs or alcohol. Considering oneself to be a burden on others is a sign of having chronic low-esteem.

34. A) Face the patient in good lighting
During a clinical interview with a patient with hearing loss, the nurse should face the patient in good lighting. This helps the patient in lipreading. The rate of speaking of the nurse should be slow. Also, the nurse should avoid looking down while speaking. Speaking at a high volume and not looking directly at the patient make lipreading difficult for the patient. The nurse should provide written instructions in addition to explaining the instructions verbally before closing the clinical interview.

35. D) Advise against Saint-John's-wort due to interactions with the prescribed medication
Saint-John's-wort, when taken with selective serotonin reuptake inhibitors (SSRIs), can increase the risk of serotonin syndrome. Therefore, the nurse will advise against the use of Saint-John's-wort. Simply providing education on the safe use of herbal supplements would not offer the patient the accurate and important information they need when taking a supplement that would interact with prescribed medication; advising on proper dosages would also not be appropriate. The patient would not be instructed to stop the prescribed medication without further assessment. While Saint-John's-wort does have interactions with other prescribed medications, it is not known to directly impact mental health symptoms.

36. D) Implementing the DASH diet and monthly monitoring sessions
Research supports the DASH diet, or a similar nutritional program, and activity for weight reduction for patients with different types of weight gain, including medication-related weight gain. Weight management monitoring should be scheduled at least once monthly. It is not necessary to refer the patient to a weight-loss specialist at this time. The nurse should never suggest stopping a prescribed medication. Adding combination herbal supplements is not an appropriate intervention because many herbs have serious interactive effects with prescribed medications.

37. D) Negotiate with the patient to reduce herb usage while discussing a possible trial of prescribed medication
One way the nurse can help a patient who is highly reluctant to stop using a harmful substance is negotiation. The nurse can try to negotiate with the patient about repatterning the usage of the herb so that they can come to a mutual understanding. Negotiation can also be used to introduce a trial of prescribed medication. The nurse will not encourage the patient to continue using the herb in the same manner without an attempt to reduce or discontinue the herb. The nurse should not use intimidation to persuade the patient to stop using the herb. Demanding a behavior change is rarely helpful and should not be the approach the nurse uses.

38. A) Cognitive behavioral therapy

The patient shows symptoms of attention deficit hyperactivity disorder (ADHD). Cognitive behavioral therapy is highly recommended because it helps in management of everyday tasks and management of time, and it improves productivity. Removing the child from school should be a last resort. Patients with ADHD should strictly avoid honey and white rice in the diet, as these may worsen ADHD symptoms. Donepezil is also recommended for ADHD but should not be given to patients younger than 8 years.

39. A) Pauses collecting the history and politely asks the patient which behavior was offensive

Asking which behavior has offended the patient helps to build rapport between the patient and the nurse and helps to regain the patient's trust. Offering reassurance to the patient may be warranted, but the nurse would determine the cause of offense before moving on to the next question. Asking culturally insensitive questions is a mistake that any nurse can make, but it does not mean that the nurse will stop the interview and turn the patient's care over to someone else. The nurse should ask the patient about the patient's culture because this will help the nurse to know more about the culture and to avoid causing the patient unintentional pain. It will also show the patient that the nurse has a desire to know more about the patient's culture.

40. B) Request that hospital security accompany the nurse into the patient interview

The patient is exhibiting behavior indicative of intermittent explosive disorder. The priority is to ensure safety by asking security to be present during the patient interview. Placing the patient in handcuffs or restraining the patient in the bed would not be the appropriate intervention at this time. The family may need to be contacted, but this would occur after the nurse establishes a safe environment and only if the patient could not provide the information.

41. D) Step away from the patient and call for security to be present for the rest of the assessment

The most appropriate action would be to step away from the patient, go to the door or phone, and call for assistance. The nurse would not leave the patient alone because he may injure himself or possibly leave the facility. Speaking calmly and softly is an appropriate way to communicate with the patient, but if feeling unsafe, the nurse should trust their instincts and not engage the patient because he may become aggressive.

42. D) Collect a blood specimen from the patient for thiamine level
Thiamine and niacin levels are low in patients with alcohol use disorders due to poor eating habits and malabsorption of minerals. Severe thiamine deficiency can cause delirium, confusion, and hallucinations and should be treated with intravenous thiamine. Physical restraints should be a last resort. Providing education on proper weaning is not an appropriate action while the patient is disoriented. Administering naloxone would not be appropriate for this patient because naloxone is used in the case of opioid overdose.

43. A) Continue the process to admit the patient according to the court order
The patient is exhibiting behavior that supports emergency commitment. The appropriate step would be to follow through with the admission so the patient can be further evaluated and treated. A second opinion may be requested later, but at this time the nurse must follow the court order. It would not be appropriate to discuss alternatives to an involuntary commitment. The nurse should not be dishonest about the admission.

44. A) The patient and the family can benefit from functional family therapy
In a situation where there is conflict within the family unit, the best treatment plan for optimal recovery is to treat the family as a whole with functional family therapy. Conflict in the family has been determined to be a cause of relapse and failure to recover in patients with substance use disorder. When possible, the family should be addressed as a unit. Individual needs such as parenting classes would be identified through family therapy. While it is important for the patient to discontinue drug use, this is only one step in the treatment and recovery process. The patient may benefit from being placed in another home that is a hostility-free environment, but that is a determination to be made after further evaluation and with input from the patient.

45. B) AUDIT
Alcohol Use Disorders Identification Test (AUDIT) is a widely used tool to determine the severity of alcohol use and is especially beneficial when patients self-identify that there may be a problem. The tool can be administered by either the nurse or the patient and is an early identifier of alcohol use disorder (AUD). The CAGE assessment tool is an excellent initial tool if the nurse suspects alcohol use may be an issue, but it is brief and used to identify alcohol use that the patient may not report. The T-ACE screening tool is specific to patients who are pregnant, and screening, brief intervention, referral to treatment (SBIRT) is a screening and intervention approach used to determine and treat high-risk behaviors that may lead to AUD. This approach integrates screening, assessment, and intervention and is a tool that can be used alone or with other tools.

46. B) Concrete operational

The child is in the concrete operational stage at around age 7 to 11 years. It is the third stage of intellectual development. This stage brings an increasing orientation to the reality-based world and more organized, coherent mental structures that allow for internal, rather than action-oriented, problem-solving. Children in this age-group are unable to use deductive reasoning. Thinking is concrete and lacks moral reasoning abilities. The formal operational stage is present from age 11 years through adolescence. During this stage, there is a shift to higher level abstract thinking and hypothetical deductive reasoning, and patients are able to reason and change their thinking. The preoperational stage (from age 18 months to 7 years) is marked by object permanence and imitation. Thinking is egocentric. These children view the world from their point of view and ask "why" questions. They cannot reason, use logic, or combine ideas. They have trouble assessing between quantity and appearance. In the sensorimotor stage (birth to 18 months), the child actively constructs information about the world via physical explorations and actions. They lack object permanence.

47. D) SBIRT

SBIRT (screening, brief intervention, referral to treatment) is a screening and intervention approach used to determine and treat high-risk behaviors that may lead to alcohol use disorder (AUD). This approach integrates screening, assessment, and intervention and is a tool that can be used alone or with other tools. It is an initial screening for patients who have not self-reported alcohol use. The Alcohol Use Disorders Identification Test (AUDIT) is a widely used tool to determine the severity of alcohol use and is especially beneficial when patients self-identify that there may be a problem. The tool can be administered by either the nurse or the patient. The CAGE assessment tool is an excellent initial tool if the nurse suspects alcohol use may be an issue. The assessment is brief and is used to identify a patient's alcohol use that the patient may not report. The T-ACE screening tool is specific to patients who are pregnant.

48. B) Shared decision-making

Shared decision-making forms the basis of any therapeutic alliance. Soliciting the patient's perspective through shared discussion around decision-making begins the therapeutic alliance. Setting limits or boundaries is a factor in the relationship, but the initial session priority is forming the therapeutic alliance. Self-identification as the expert is a paternalistic approach that diminishes the patient's power to be capable of self-determination. Creating a safety plan may be appropriate in cases where suicidal risks exists, but without the presence of a therapeutic alliance, the patient may not feel safe enough to disclose.

49. A) Glutamate
Glutamate is the universal excitatory neurotransmitter. It is involved with kindling, seizure disorders, and possibly bipolar disorder. The universal inhibitory neurotransmitter is GABA. Acetylcholine is cholinergic and is not associated with kindling, seizure disorders, or bipolar disorder. Glycine is also an inhibitory neurotransmitter.

50. D) Literacy level of reference material
Any time reference material is provided, it is recommended that the material be written at an eighth grade reading level because that is the average reading level of an adult in the United States. The age of the attendees does not automatically indicate their reading level. The length of the reference is irrelevant if the attendees cannot read and comprehend the material. Decisions regarding reference material should be based on the attendees' needs, not the preferences of the staff.

51. B) Antipsychotic-induced extrapyramidal symptoms
Poor metabolizers of *CYP2D6* may develop higher levels of antipsychotic drugs, resulting in adverse effects such as extrapyramidal symptoms (EPS) and hyperprolactinemia. Multiple studies have shown a relationship between dysfunctional *CYP2D6* variants and antipsychotic-induced EPS, especially tardive dyskinesia. Inadequate dosing is a risk for patients who are ultrarapid metabolizers. They require higher doses; without alteration in dose, ultrarapid metabolizers may experience decrease or loss in efficacy. Poor metabolizers are not at risk for gene–drug interactions.

52. B) Communication
The priority at this time is to assess the patient's ability to communicate and their ability to understand the information that is being given to them. Language barriers prevent the exchange of accurate information, leading to an inaccurate plan of care. Clear communication must be established before the nurse can assess other factors such gender identity, risk factors, and citizenship.

53. A) "Are you using any type of birth control at this time?"
Contraception is an important item to assess with lithium therapy because lithium can have significant effects on a fetus. Patients who are able to become pregnant should have a pregnancy test prior to administration, and the risks associated with pregnancy should be discussed; contraception should be encouraged. While some visual symptoms such as blurry vision can occur with lithium, this is not related to damage to the eye, so the date of the last eye exam is not relevant. Due to the potential renal consequences, patients should be advised to significantly limit ibuprofen intake; acetaminophen would be the preferred medication for pain. Identifying a history of sleepwalking is important in all situations, but it is not specific to the effects of lithium.

54. A) Mood
Lamotrigine (Lamictal) can be prescribed for a number of conditions including seizure disorders, neuropathic pain, migraine headaches, and bipolar disorder. When treating bipolar disorder, lamotrigine is used to help stabilize mood; it does not have a direct effect on attention span or sleep. Lamotrigine is not prescribed for tremors.

55. D) The nurse should ask about other inventions that were tried prior to administering the alprazolam
Alprazolam (Xanax) is used as a short-term treatment for generalized anxiety disorder while waiting for other long-term medications, such as SSRIs, to be effective. Alprazolam should be used sparingly and only on an as-needed basis. To ensure cautious use, the nurse should ask about nonpharmaceutical interventions, such as breathing exercises, before administering a pharmaceutical treatment such as a benzodiazepine. Because alprazolam is indicated for short-term use, the initial treatment plan would not include an increasing dose of the medication over the course of several months. The administered dose should be the lowest dose needed to achieve the desired effect; there is no set target dose. For some patients, alprazolam is used sparingly for a longer period of time, but this is done as an adjunct to SSRIs, not as a replacement. The abuse potential that is associated with alprazolam is the primary reason for limiting the medication to short-term, as-needed use. If abuse is suspected, interventions such as random pill counts may be implemented; however, planned benzodiazepine blood testing is not used.

56. A) "To be completely honest, it is not clear exactly how the medication works."
While lithium is the gold standard for the treatment of dipolar disorder, the exact mechanism of action is still grossly unknown, and the nurse should provide transparent information to the patient. Selective serotonin reuptake inhibitors (SSRIs) work by inhibiting serotonin uptake, while serotonin and norepinephrine reuptake inhibitors (SNRIs) regulate norepinephrine and serotonin. Second-generation antipsychotics modify dopamine and serotonin levels.

57. C) Pseudoephedrine (Sudafed)
Benztropine (Cogentin) is an anticholinergic drug that can be used to treat Parkinson disease. Patients who are prescribed this medication should avoid other anticholinergic medications, such as pseudoephedrine, as they can intensify the anticholinergic effects of benztropine, producing dangerous effects. Polyethylene glycol does not interact with the prescribed medication and would be recommended to treat the common side effect of constipation. There are no medication interactions between benztropine, acetaminophen, and/or ondansetron; these medications can be safely taken together.

58. A) Death
The boxed warning associated with antipsychotics is an increased risk of death when the medication is administered to older adult patients with dementia-related psychosis; chlorpromazine is a first-generation antipsychotic medication. Antipsychotics do not increase the risk of dementia or stroke. An increased risk of suicidal ideation, primarily in adolescents and young adults, is the boxed warning that is associated with antidepressants.

59. A) One hour prior to the scheduled activity
The onset of immediate-release carbidopa/levodopa (Sinemet) is less than 1 hour, and the half-life is less than 2 hours. To facilitate movement control during the physical activity, the nurse should administer a dose of the medication 1 hour prior to the scheduled activity. Administration of the medication 4 hours, 8 hours, or the night before would not be therapeutic because the effectiveness of the immediate-release medication would be minimal to none at that time; those time frames are more appropriate for extended-release medications.

60. B) Perform a complete respiratory assessment

Loxapine (Adasuve) can cause severe bronchospasms that have the potential to lead to respiratory distress or respiratory arrest. The most important action for the nurse to complete is a respiratory assessment to evaluate for possible bronchospasms. At times, a second antipsychotic may be needed, but the full effects of the administered medication would not be seen in 15 minutes. There is no drug level associated with loxapine (Adasuve). A full set of vital signs can be obtained as a general survey for patient safety but does not assess for adverse reactions that are specific to the medication.

61. A) "The dose will be increased weekly until the target dose is met."

Memantine (Namenda) is used to treat Alzheimer disease. The medication is started as a low, once-a-day dose that is increased weekly until the target dose is achieved. The patient does not have to return to the clinic for every dose increase, and 4 weeks is too long of an interval for medication titration. Increasing the dose every other day is too rapid and can cause adverse medication effects. The ability to draw a clock is used as a screening tool for cognitive impairment, but it does not measure disease progress; the dose increase would not be based on the outcomes of an individual screening tool.

62. D) Assign distancing anytime the patient is outside of their room

The nurse should explain the basics of illness transmission and assign distancing as a measure of reducing illness transmission. Because masks often have strings, they are not traditionally allowed on patient units. Asking the other patients to wear masks would not be appropriate due to the previously described mask components. While medical illnesses are not as prevalent in mental health facilities, those illnesses are still present.

63. B) Conduct a role-play session with the patient that mimics the observed behavior

Before assuming that the patient is purposely disregarding the instructions provided, the nurse should ensure that the patient understood what was taught. This can be assessed using role-play. Use of a pharmaceutical intervention should come after nonpharmaceutical measures have been attempted. Restricting the patient's privileges without correcting the behavior does not lead to long-term resolution. Making negative statements that imply the nurse is disappointed in the patient is not appropriate; if necessary, the nurse can communicate that they are disappointed in the patient's behavior, but not the patient themself.

64. C) Make an announcement asking all available hospital staff to report to the unit
Prior to initiating physical restraints, the nurse can implement a "show of force" where additional hospital staff members present to the unit to assist with the emergency patient situation. At times this can de-escalate patient behavior. If the show of force is ineffective or if the situation worsens, additional assistance is already present. Allowing the patient to go to another unit during a time in which they are potentially harmful to others would create a safety issue. The nurse may call the provider to request a change to the route of administration of the medication; however, this is not something the nurse can do independently. Unless the presence of the current technician is a triggering agent, there is no reason to swap the mental health technicians.

65. A) Review the monthly stool diary
The co-occurrence of encopresis and chronic constipation is common. Parents and caregivers should be advised to keep a monthly stool diary that will provide significant insight into the recent stool pattern. The stool pattern is a major factor in determining the current state of the condition. At times a digital rectal exam is needed; however, this would not be the first step because it is an invasive action. A change in abdominal circumference and weight would not be present unless constipation was very severe, which would present with other severe symptoms that are not currently noted.

66. A) "Can you describe the current state of the patient's personal matters?"
Generally speaking, a conservatorship removes decision-making capabilities from the patient and places this authority with another individual. This only occurs if the patient is unable to manage their personal affairs due to a medical or mental health condition. To determine if a conservatorship is indicated, the nurse should assess the state of the patient's personal matters to determine if the patient is appropriately maintaining. A conservatorship is a legal mandate; therefore, patient consent is not needed. While spending habits would be evidence of poor financial decision-making, this one factor could not determine the need for a conservatorship. Violent outbursts or episodes of self-harm would warrant evaluation for inpatient treatment.

67. D) "Can you tell me about your sexual encounters recently?"
Evaluating sexual behavior is multifactorial. The best method for assessing the patient's recent behavior is asking an open-ended question that allows the patient to provide the initial information; the nurse can elaborate on the information provided by the patient. Asking about the number of sexual partners provides limited information because having just one partner does not mean the concerning behaviors are not present. Even if the patient is having appropriate sex with their spouse, asking about this does not assess for sexual activity outside of the relationship. STI testing is recommended in this situation; however, completing the testing is not a reflection of the state of the behavior.

68. C) "What made you decide to volunteer at at flower nursery?"
As with any phobia, the treatment of agoraphobia involves the patient learning to cope with the condition, which includes avoiding triggers and identifying situations that would be therapeutic. By asking the patient what made them decide to volunteer at the flower nursery, the nurse is able to assess the patient's ability to identify appropriate situations. The patient has already stated that they are ready to move forward, so asking again would not be appropriate; the nurse should ask questions that provide more substantive information. Patients progress at different rates, so the amount of time in therapy does not automatically indicate readiness. It is not mandatory that the patient disclose their mental health diagnosis, and disclosure to a new employer does not necessarily mean the patient is or is not ready to volunteer.

69. B) Establish when the symptoms initially began
Dysfunctional grief is defined by the length of time the symptoms have been present and the severity of the symptoms. To establish if dysfunctional grieving is present, the nurse should begin by determining when the symptoms started so a timeline is understood. Directly assessing the patient's relationship with other children would not provide insight into the patient's journey in the grief process. If the patient's behaviors were concerning for a mood disorder, a screening tool would be administered, but this is not a standard tool used in evaluating grief. Goals should be set after the nurse determines the patient's current state.

70. D) There has been one identifiable episode of mania
Bipolar I disorder requires that the *DSM-5* criteria for at least one manic episode must be met. A depressive episode is not required for a diagnosis of bipolar I disorder. Hospitalization is not required for all manic episodes and is therefore not a criterion for bipolar I disorder. Although the lifetime suicide risk for individuals with bipolar disorder is 15 times higher than that for the general population, history of suicide attempt is not a criterion for either bipolar I or bipolar II disorder.

71. C) Psychomotor agitation

Psychomotor agitation is one of nine symptoms listed as *DSM-5* criteria A for major depressive disorder. It is exhibited through rubbing or pulling of the skin and/or clothing. Pacing is a key manifestation, as is inability to be still or fidgeting. While restlessness is found in generalized anxiey disorder, worry and fatigue are key features, which are not present in this patient. Likewise, those with obsessive-compulsive disorder have irritability and agitation, but this is due to an inability to control their environment. Patients with obsessive-compulsive disorder will have obtrusive thoughts that involve rituals and/or numbers, such as washing their hands for a certain amount of time. Atypical features of depression include mood reactivity, significant weight gain/increase in appetite, leaden paralysis, hypersomnia, or interpersonal rejection.

72. A) Evidence of mania

Bipolar I disorder requires that the *DSM-5* criteria for at least one manic episode must be met. This is the factor that differentiates bipolar I from bipolar II disorder. History of suicide attempt, psychiatric hospitalization, and episode(s) of depression do not distinguish bipolar I from bipolar II disorder.

73. D) Weight loss

The symptoms of hyperthyroidism may mimic signs and symptoms of a manic episode or severe anxiety. These symptoms include increased pulse, fine tremor, heat intolerance with excessive sweating, weight loss, hyperverbal speech, exaggerated startle response, menstrual irregularities, muscle weakness, and exophthalmos. Weight gain can be seen in hypothyroidism, which often mimics symptoms of depression. Abdominal pain and dry mouth are not specific to hyperthyroidism, but they may be seen in lithium toxicity, which could be present if the patient has been taking lithium. However, patient treatment has not yet been initiated.

74. B) Cold intolerance

The symptoms of hypothyroidism are commonly mistaken for depression. Symptoms of hypothyroidism include apathy, weight gain, thin and dry hair, cold intolerance, facial puffiness, and slowed thinking. Therefore, it is important for the nurse to rule this condition out prior to starting a patient on an antidepressant. Tachycardia is commonly seen in hyperthyroidism, which often mimics anxiety or mania. Difficulty sleeping and pruritis are also associated with hyperthyroidism.

75. A) Spina bifida at birth

Spina bifida is a common neuronal defect seen in neonates who have been exposed in utero to valproate (Depakote) or carbamazepine (Tegretol), both of which are well-known neuronal teratogens used to treat seizure disorders. Cleft palate is not a neurologic disorder and may be seen with various medications given in utero, including lamotrigine (Lamictal), a neuroleptic medication that can be used to treat seizures. Ebstein anomaly is a cardiac abnormality seen in patients exposed to lithium in utero; lithium is used to treat mood disorders and may be used adjunctly in the treatment of depression. Neonatal withdrawal syndrome may occur with controlled substances or other drugs such as selective serotonin reuptake inhibitors (SSRIs), which are used to treat depression. However, SSRIs are not considered neurologic teratogens.

76. D) Lamotrigine (Lamictal)

Stevens–Johnson syndrome is life-threatening epidermal necrolysis that can occur in patients taking lamotrigine. The risk of Stevens–Johnson syndrome is increased with concomitant use of valproate. Concurrent use of lamotrigine and valproate should be avoided if at all possible. Lithium carbonate, lurasidone, and cariprazine are used in the treatment of bipolar depression; however, risk of Stevens–Johnson syndrome is not a concern with these medications.

77. C) Agranulocytosis

Carbamazepine is an anticonvulsant agent often used as an off-label treatment for bipolar disorder. Among the adverse reactions to carbamazepine are blood dyscrasias such as agranulocytosis and aplastic anemia. Symptoms of agranulocytosis include sore throat, fever, and oral and perianal ulcerations. Neuroleptic malignant syndrome is associated with use of antipsychotics. Serotonin syndrome is caused by use of antidepressants and other medications concurrently that increase levels of serotonin. Anticonvulsant intoxication or an overdose of carbamazepine would present with delirium or psychosis.

78. D) Imipramine (Tofranil)

Tricyclic antidepressants such as imipramine (Tofranil) have a risk for cardiac conduction effects. Although all selective serotonin reuptake inhibitors and serotonin antagonist and reuptake inhibitors, such as escitalopram, vilazodone, and trazodone, can lengthen QT intervals, it is usually in combination with an antipsychotic medication.

79. B) Adjust the time of the administration of the SSRI

Adjustment of the timing of administration of the SSRI may resolve unwanted daytime sleepiness and should be the first step to manage this side effect. Changing the medication may be considered only after all other interventions have failed. Caffeine intake should not be a recommended daily intervention. Difficulty with sleep is a common symptom for patients with mood disorders, but polyphamacy is to be avoided whenever possible and implemented only after other interventions have failed.

80. D) Participating in interprofessional meetings about treatment

The nurse role includes participation on interprofessional teams, and adherence to ethical standards of practice includes addressing risks, benefits, and outcomes for each patient. In compliance with ethical standards regarding patient confidentiality, providers may not speak with family members without patient consent. It is a breach of confidentiality to review records that are not for the nurse's patients. Only direct caregivers may access patient information without patient consent. In order to maintain adherence to ethical practice standards, all information shared between providers must be exchanged per the patient's consent. Medical records cannot be released unless under subpoena, even after patient death.

81. A) Participating on a hospital committee to ensure that patients with substance use disorders have equal access to care

According to the American Psychiatric Nurses Association (APNA), a core competency for ethical practice includes advocating for access and parity of services for mental health problems, psychiatric disorders, and substance use disorder. Participation in interprofessional teams to discuss risks, benefits, and outcomes adheres to ethical practice standards. Scope of practice involves informing the patient of all aspects of their care, including their right to be discharged against medical advice when their hospitalization is voluntary. According to the APNA, ethical competency also includes reporting illegal, incompetent, or impaired practices. The patient's confidentiality can be breached without the patient's permission when the patient has revealed a determined intention to injure or kill a specific person. It does not matter where the potential victim lives.

82. D) May cause activation of suicidal thoughts

Activation of suicidal thoughts is a boxed warning on all antidepressants, indicating the increased risk of suicidal thoughts in children and adolescents. Although dosage, risk of serotonin syndrome, and time until medication takes effect should also be discussed, patient education on the possibility of suicidal thoughts takes precedence because of the high risk of death.

83. A) Sleep hygiene

The patient is presenting with symptoms of insomnia. The nurse should educate the patient regarding sleep hygiene practices and identify modifiable factors that may be affecting the patient's sleep. A mood record, Patient Health Questionnaire–9 (PHQ-9), and General Anxiety Disorder–7 (GAD-7) screening tool would be important assessment tools and points of psychoeducation to use during an initial evaluation; however, the patient's primary report of symptoms should lead the nurse to suspect insomnia, so the priority is to assess sleep hygiene.

84. D) The patient should avoid consuming foods that are high in tyramine

Phenelzine is a monoamine oxidase inhibitor (MAOI) used in treatment-resistant depression. A life-threatening side effect of this medication is hypertensive crisis, which can occur when the patient consumes food and drink high in tyramine, such as smoked meats, fish, aged cheese, beer, red wine, and fermented foods. A slow titration is not necessary with phenelzine, and neither is a slow taper when discontinuing because the drug wears off slowly over 2 to 3 weeks. Although phenelzine may cause sedation, this side effect is rare because phenelzine is usually activating; moreover, increased sedation is not a life-threatening adverse effect.

85. A) Persistent nausea and vomiting

Lithium toxicity can occur with lithium levels above 1.5. Toxicity ranges from mild to severe, with symptoms including, but not limited to, persistent nausea and vomiting, abdominal pain, ataxia, tremors, blurred vision, delirium, syncope, and coma. Constant diarrhea, hyperthermia, and uncontrolled shivering are not signs of lithium toxicity but of serotonin syndrome, which may occur with concurrent use of lithium and an antidepressant.

86. B) Smoked salmon

A hypertensive crisis occurs when MAOIs are taken with tyramine-containing foods, such as smoked fish, aged cheeses, cured meats, organ meats, red wine, beer, and fermented foods such as sauerkraut. Ripe bananas, chicken breast, and vodka do not contain tyramine.

87. A) Primary hypothyroidism

Primary hypothyroidism occurs when free T4 is decreased and TSH levels are elevated in response to the low T4. It occurs due to destruction of the thyroid gland, as in autoimmune disease, surgery, and radioiodine or radiation therapy. It can also occur as a result of low intake of iodine; however, that is now rare due to the addition of iodine to table salt. In secondary hypothyroidism, the pituitary gland fails and both TSH and free T4 are low. Hyperthyroidism and acute thyroiditis both present with elevated free T4 levels.

88. B) Serum creatinine of 2.0 mg/dL

A rare adverse effect of long-term lithium use is nephrotoxicity. This is indicated by serum creatinine of greater than 1.3 mg/dL (normal levels are 0.6 to 1.3 mg/dL) and a glomerular filtration rate of less than 60. A glomerular filtration rate of 90 is normal, as is free thyroxine of 0.8 ng/dL and thyroid-stimulating hormone of 5.0 mU/L.

89. C) 6 months

A patient with GAD must present with anxiety and worry and experience at least three of the following symptoms for 6 months or more to be diagnosed with GAD: excess worry, restlessness, fatigue, muscle tension, and decreased sleep and concentration.

90. B) 2 weeks

Although the symptoms of major depression can last for years, to meet the criteria for a diagnosis of major depressive disorder, a patient must have five of the following symptoms for at least 2 weeks: depressed mood, lack of interest or pleasure (anhedonia), weight loss or weight gain, increased or decreased activity, feelings of hopelessness/worthlessness or guilt, fatigue/loss of energy, insomnia or hypersomnia, diminished ability to think or concentrate, and/or recurring thoughts of death or suicide. At least one of those symptoms must be depressed mood or anhedonia.

91. B) Thiamine level

Wernicke–Korsakoff syndrome is a condition resulting from depleted thiamine related to chronic alcohol abuse. Wernicke encephalopathy is an acute presentation, whereas Korsakoff syndrome is a chronic impairment in memory and anterograde amnesia in an alert and responsive patient. Alcohol misuse should be assessed in all older adults presenting with dementia. Complete blood count, basic metabolic panel, and folic acid level tests are appropriate for a patient presenting with confusion; however, only a thiamine level would assess for the chronic condition of Korsakoff syndrome.

92. B) "How long do your symptoms last?"

To differentiate between bipolar I and bipolar II disorders is to differentiate between a manic and a hypomanic episode. This is determined by the duration of the symptoms. Bipolar I would indicate manic symptoms that last for 7 days or longer, whereas bipolar II (hypomanic) symptoms last 4 to 6 days. A manic episode can also be characterized by the presence of psychosis or of symptoms so severe that the patient requires hospitalization, regardless of the duration of symptoms. Asking if the patient feels unstoppable, if they are easily distracted, or if they feel depressed would not differentiate between bipolar I and bipolar II because these symptoms are found in both disorders.

93. A) "Do your symptoms occur episodically?"

Bipolar disorder and ADHD share common traits such as rapid speech, racing thoughts, distractibility, and reduced need for sleep. In order to differentiate these symptoms as bipolar disorder or ADHD symptomology, the nurse must ask if the presenting symptoms occur episodically. With bipolar disorder, the symptoms would be present only periodically during the manic episode, and when the patient switches to a depressed or euthymic state, the manic symptoms would resolve. In the case of a comorbid presentation, the nurse may ask if the symptoms worsen during a distinct period of time, which may indicate that the symptoms are presenting during a manic episode. The questions "Are you easily distracted?" "Do your friends say you talk too fast?" and "Would you say your symptoms are troubling?" would not differentiate bipolar disorder from ADHD because these symptoms are present in both disorders.

94. B) Bipolar I disorder

The patient is exhibiting signs consistent with a manic episode of a bipolar I presentation. To differentiate between bipolar I and bipolar II disorders is to differentiate between a manic and a hypomanic episode. These are typically differentiated by the duration of the symptoms. Bipolar I is indicated by manic symptoms that last for 7 days or longer, whereas bipolar II (hypomanic) symptoms last for 4 to 6 days. However, a manic episode can also be characterized by the presence of psychosis, such as hearing voices, or of symptoms so severe that the patient requires hospitalization, regardless of the duration of symptoms. Both bipolar I and bipolar II diagnostic criteria must also meet the criteria for major depressive disorder; however, the addition of the manic symptoms justifies a bipolar I diagnosis. A brief psychotic episode is a period of psychosis that lasts less than 30 days but that cannot be better explained by a major depressive episode or bipolar disorder.

95. C) Enroll in a psychology course at the local community college
Part of recovery is to make healthy choices and lifestyle changes that help an individual to reach their highest potential. Enrolling in a course is a step toward making positive changes. While it is a good idea to reflect, an essential part of recovery is to make changes, and too much time spent reflecting misses a crucial element of the recovery process. While obtaining a job is a positive step forward, a position at a distillery or a pain clinic poses a risk for relapse due to the high likelihood of being exposed to alcohol or pain medication.

96. C) Ensure that the patient feels safe and secure
The healing process and interactions with the patient should start by building rapport and ensuring that the patient feels safe to assist with the stabilization process, to be followed by assessment of the need for further crisis interventions. A patient is more likely to be open and honest when they feel safe and trust their practitioner. The nurse might later provide background, discuss the therapeutic process, obtain history, and discuss treatment options, but assessing safety must come before anything else.

97. A) CAGE questionnaire
The CAGE questionnaire is a quick screening tool that can assess alcoholism in a patient. A positive response to two or more of the questions increases the likelihood that the patient might struggle with alcoholism, and the nurse should then perform a further evaluation. The Clinical Institute Withdrawal Assessment (CIWA) scale is a tool that is used to assess a patient who is experiencing alcohol withdrawal. The Hamilton Rating Scale for Depression is a tool used to evaluate a patient's depression complaints and is not specific to alcohol usage. Referring to the *DSM-5* can help target the reported findings and assist with questioning, but it is not a specific screening tool for alcoholism and instead assists with determining if the patient meets the criteria for a particular mental illness.

98. A) ACE
The Adverse Childhood Experiences (ACE) Scale can play a role in identifying a patient's likelihood of suffering from diseases, mental health issues, and poorer outcomes. Recognizing the score early on helps guide implementation of healthy interventions into the treatment plan to improve patient outcomes and assist with the development of resilience and recovery from these adverse experiences. The Mini-Mental State Examination (MMSE) assesses patients' cognition and overall cognitive abilities to look for any signs of dementia. It is usually performed in the older adult population. The Child Attachment Interview (CAI) looks into what things are like in a family from the patient's point of view to help the interviewer better understand the patient. The YMRS is the Young Mania Rating Scale, used to assess the patient's severity of manic symptoms.

99. A) Amitriptyline (Elavil)

Amitriptyline is contraindicated in patients who recently experienced myocardial infarction and the resultant risk of developing cardiovascular arrhythmias, heart failure, QT prolongation, and other serious cardiovascular complications. Sertraline and fluoxetine have proved cardiovascular safety in patients suffering from depression following a myocardial infarction. While there is limited information on cardiovascular complications, lamotrigine is not contraindicated, although it should be used with caution. As with all other medications, careful consideration of the patient's history and current medicines, as well as knowledge of the risks, benefits, indications, and contraindications of drugs, is essential in the prescriptive process.

100. B) Guilt

The "G" in CAGE stands for Guilt and asks the patient if they have ever felt guilty about their drinking. Gluttony, greed, and gauge are not aspects of the CAGE questionnaire.

101. B) Has pinpoint pupils

Patients who are acutely intoxicated with opioids may have pinpoint pupils, display slurred speech, be sedated, and, if recently injected, may have track marks or new injection sites that are noticeable during the assessment. Although sedation can be present with opioid intoxication, the patient appearing tired but easily arousable would not, by itself, warrant a toxicology screening. Similarly, a disheveled appearance is insufficient grounds for a toxicology screening; there may be many reasons for the appearance that are unrelated to substance use. Long-term opioid use, in general, can lead to the development of constipation; however, there are several other reasons that the patient might be reporting constipation. The nurse would require more information and further assessment to determine if the constipation is caused by opioid use.

102. B) "Do you ever feel you should cut down on your drinking?"

The "C" in the CAGE mnemonic refers to whether the patient ever feels the need to cut down on their drinking. This question is used during screening as an initial nonthreatening inquiry. Asking if the patient enjoys drinking is not included in the CAGE questionnaire. Asking about the decision to cut down or if the patient thinks they have a drinking problem are good follow-up questions that can be useful after the initial screening but are not included in the CAGE questionnaire.

103. D) Spends more time discussing the patient's religion and how it may impact decision-making
Cultural competence is demonstrated by the nurse's effort to seek a better understanding of the patient's religion and how it impacts their decision-making. Telling the patient that they have to take the medication to feel better or having a person of another religious background discuss the treatment plan with the patient does not demonstrate cultural competence or understanding. The nurse's immediately resorting to documenting refusal of treatment is not conducive to understanding or helping the patient.

104. B) Feeling she has self-worth despite her family relationships
Self-differentiation is the level at which an individual's self-worth is not dependent on external relationships. Enmeshment in family boundaries demonstrates lack of self-differentiation because of the value external relationships hold in such patterns. Continued low self-worth demonstrates lack of self-differentiation. Self-identity is not a factor when determining self-differentiation.

105. A) Ensuring that the patient has a trusted family member with whom to discuss the treatment plan
The nurse has a duty to advocate for patients, which includes actions such as having trusted family members to ensure understanding of the treatment plan. Failure to obtain patient consent and disregarding information about the patient's healthcare power of attorney demonstrate lack of advocacy for the patient. Education, including allowing time for questions, is a significant component of advocacy to ensure that the patient is able to make informed decisions about treatment.

106. B) Returns to stability despite continuing dysfunction
Homeostasis indicates the family's achievement of stability, despite dysfunction. Continuing with maladaptive communication and previous behavior patterns suggests no change in the family system, with continuing negative outcomes. Less effective communication between family members demonstrates a worsening outcome for the family system, which is not congruent with achievement of homeostasis/stability.

107. B) Family structure, subsystems, and boundaries
Family structure, subsystems, boundaries, and enmeshment are key concepts of structural family therapy. Reframing and paradoxical interventions are key concepts of strategic therapy. Homeostasis and feedback loops are key concepts of strategic family therapy. Emotions and attachment styles are discussed in emotionally focused family therapy.

108. A) Level achieved when one's self-worth is not dependent on external relationships
Self-differentiation is a key concept of family systems therapy and is the level achieved when one's self-worth is not dependent on external relationships. Self-differentiation does not involve differentiating problematic traits; it is independent in nature. Relabeling of problematic self-fulfilling behaviors to have more positive meaning is an example of reframing. Attempting to break contact between self and family members is called cutting off, not self-differentiation.

109. B) The problem and the sequence of interactions that maintain the problem
Strategic family therapy is problem focused, and techniques include those that focus on changing the sequence of interactions that is causing the problem. Focusing on family structure to effectively manage problems is important when using structural family therapy. Focusing on self-confrontation of each family member is important in an individual therapy approach with existential therapy. Self-differentiation is a key concept in family systems theory.

110. B) Precontemplation, contemplation, preparation, action, and maintenance
The transtheoretical model of change includes the stages of precontemplation, contemplation, preparation, action, and maintenance. Freezing, unfreezing, and action are components of Kurt Lewin's change theory, which does not include contemplation, transition, or maintenance. Plan, do, study, and act are stages of the plan-do-study-act (PDSA) model, but maintain is not a stage in this model, and it is unrelated to the transtheoretical model of change.

111. B) States that their marijuana use is not a big deal
During the precontemplation phase, the individual does not identify problematic behavior and does not demonstrate readiness for change. The patient stating that they plan to stop next month and acknowledging that marijuana use is a problem show that the patient is ready to change and is planning interventions for change in the near future. The patient's agreement to reduce marijuana use before the next visit demonstrates action that the patient is willing to take to reduce problematic behavior.

112. B) "My drinking is a problem, and I'm thinking about how to improve in the next few months."
According to the transtheoretical model of change, in the contemplation phase, the individual identifies problematic behavior and intends to make changes to the behavior in the near future. When the patient acknowledges alcohol misuse and wants to make changes within the next few months, the patient demonstrates readiness, which is indicative of the contemplation stage. Lack of acknowledgment of alcohol misuse, vague planning around treatment, and refusal of treatment are actions that indicate lack of readiness, or the precontemplation stage.

113. C) Schizophrenia
In patients with schizophrenia, the enhanced subcortical release of the neurotransmitter dopamine brings symptoms of delusions and hallucinations. Parkinson disease occurs as the cells "giving birth" to dopamine die. Feeling hopeless and losing motivation are some symptoms of depression, and a decrease in dopamine level enhances these issues. A lower level of dopamine is a sign of attention deficit hyperactivity disorder as well.

114. C) Hypothalamus
The suprachiasmatic nucleus is located at the hypothalamus of the brain. Its function is to maintain the regulation of the sleep–wake cycle. It is present in the hypothalamus as a cluster of many cells. This nucleus is not a part of the amygdala or the hippocampus. It is not present in the pineal gland; rather, it controls the secretion of the hormone known as melatonin from this gland.

115. B) Fatigue or loss of energy nearly every day for 2 weeks
According to the *DSM-5*, five or more symptoms of depression should be present for the same 2-week period, inclusive of fatigue or loss of energy, to meet diagnostic criteria for MDD. Three symptoms of depression over 2 weeks do not meet diagnostic criteria for MDD. While marked disinterest in activities for most of the day is a symptom of depression, symptoms must be present for at least 2 weeks to meet diagnostic criteria. Restlessness or feeling on edge is a symptom of generalized anxiety disorder, not MDD.

116. B) 50 and 125 mcg/mL
The target serum level for valproate is 50 to 125 mcg/mL. The range of 350 to 450 ng/mL is the target serum level for clozapine (Clozaril). The therapeutic range for lithium is 0.8 to 1.2 mEq/L. The range of 0.1 to 1.5 mEq/L is not a specific target range for any psychotropic medication.

117. B) 2 to 3

Antipsychotics are metabolized primarily in the liver, with metabolites excreted primarily in urine. Many metabolites are active, and peak plasma concentration usually is reached 2 to 3 hours after an oral dose.

118. C) Preparation

Self-liberation is the stage at which an individual is intending to take action. Self-liberation is found in the preparation stage. The process of consciousness-raising, dramatic belief, and reevaluation is found in precontemplation. The process of self-reevaluation is found in contemplation. The process of counter conditioning, stimulus control, and helping relationship is found in the action stage.

119. C) Materials are not written at the correct grade level

The Guidelines for Developing Patient Education Materials recommend choosing books, pamphlets, and/or brochures written at a third- to a fifth-grade level. Teaching material that is at a higher academic level does not consider the educational level of the patient. While literacy deficits can be missed, the patient was initially engaged and appeared to lose interest as the teaching continued. The initial interest from the patient suggests that they were in agreement with the discharge process. The patient was assessed in order to be able to be discharged, so it is less likely there is an active perceptual problem.

120. A) Discontinuation syndrome

Discontinuation syndrome is frequently reported with venlafaxine (Effexor). Antidepressant discontinuation syndrome can include flu-like symptoms or symptoms similar to those of panic attacks, but the most likely cause of these symptoms in this patient would be discontinuation syndrome. Sleep deprivation can cause mood changes; however, only discontinuation syndrome includes shock-like symptoms.

121. A) Increased lacrimation, rhinorrhea, and piloerection

Increased lacrimation, rhinorrhea, and piloerection are signs of early withdrawal. Typically, a patient experiencing withdrawal from short-term opioids such as heroin and morphine becomes symptomatic within 6 to 24 hours after the last dose. Pinpoint pupils and bradycardia are signs of life-threatening opioid overdose. Tonic-clonic seizures and tremors present in alcohol withdrawal. Patients withdrawing from cocaine and amphetamines experience dysthymia; vivid, unpleasant dreams; and insomnia.

122. A) Self-efficacy

Self-efficacy is confidence in one's ability to successfully perform a health behavior change. The teenage patient is confident in their ability to avoid smoking and exercise regularly, which is an example of self-efficacy. Unrealistic optimism is predicting an outcome that is not relevant or realistic; in this case, it is not unrealistic to expect to reduce the likelihood of pulmonary disease if smoking is avoided and regular exercise is performed. Self-liberation is decision-making after a process has happened. Dramatic relief refers to expressing one's feelings about a particular problem or solution.

123. B) Cognitive behavioral

Cognitive behavioral therapy would be used in this situation. This therapy addresses both the behavior and the negative thoughts of the patient. Humanistic therapy is used where self-concept is important. Interpersonal therapy is a short-term therapy of 12 to 20 weeks that is used to make current interpersonal relationships better. It works well when both participating people are ready to improve the relationship. Psychodynamic therapy is used when the past of the patient is involved.

124. C) Help patients achieve a healthier lifestyle

Helping older adults achieve a healthier, more active lifestyle is the long-term outcome for this nonprofit. The long-term outcome is the intended result of the intervention, which can be achieved by guiding older adults to participate in a healthy, active lifestyle. For the outcome to be achieved, the nonprofit includes an external condition of collaboration with a well-regarded hospital. This component is an assumption of what is needed to achieve the goal and is not the overall outcome. The number of treated patients is one of the indicators of progress toward the goal. Creating literature and spreading information about the initiative can help in reaching the goal.

125. D) Industry versus inferiority

The child has unresolved industry versus inferiority because the child has a sense of inferiority and difficulty in working and learning. The resolution of this crisis would help the child to feel confident about improving in their abilities. Unsuccessful resolution of trust versus mistrust leads to general issues relating to suspicion of people. Unsuccessful resolution of autonomy versus shame and doubt leads to fear of conflict and self-doubt. Unsuccessful resolution of initiative versus guilt leads to aggression and a sense of inadequacy.

126. C) Bipolar I

The patient's most likely diagnosis is bipolar I. Their mental state abnormalities meet the *DSM-5* criteria for bipolar I disorder (has inflated self-esteem, requires less sleep, is overtalkative, has a history of functional impairment, and has an increase in goal-directed activity). Manic symptoms have lasted for over a week. Patients with an adjustment disorder with mixed anxiety and depressed mood do not experience the severity of symptoms and loss of function this patient is experiencing. Although there is a history of stressful events, symptoms preceded these events. Steroid psychosis is categorized by the *DSM-5* as a form of substance/medication-induced psychotic disorder. The patient did not experience delusions or hallucinations after taking prednisone, and the exposure was 3 months ago. Bipolar II involves periods of hypomania; there is no history of mania. A bipolar II diagnosis requires a patient to experience at least one major depressive episode, which the patient has not experienced.

127. C) Biofeedback

Biofeedback therapy involves the use of technology and exercise that can help the patient. It can include using smartwatches to monitor changes in vital signs or doing exercises to reduce pain. Exposure therapy is used to help the patient become accustomed to a certain situation. This therapy is used for phobias and for stopping the misuse of drugs or alcohol. Aversion therapy is chosen when other measures fail to help a patient react in a certain way, and it can be used for behaviors like nail-biting. Modeling therapy involves providing a role model to the patient so that imitation can help a patient adopt the desired change.

128. B) Exposure

The patient should be treated with exposure therapy in cases of phobia. This will slowly eliminate the patient's fear and will also help reduce the anxiety. Psychoanalytical therapy is a classical theory that is not valid in many cases today. It involves looking at the dreams and childhood traumas of the patient; similarly, dream analysis would not be considered a valid therapy. Aversion therapy applies when there is substance use or when the patient is required to avoid a certain stimulus or element that has been causing harm.

129. B) Autonomy versus shame and doubt

The child is exhibiting an unresolved crisis of autonomy versus shame and doubt, generating self-doubt. Integrity versus despair is characterized by a dissatisfied sense of life. Trust versus mistrust refers to a sense of suspiciousness when it comes to trusting others. Intimacy versus isolation is characterized by emotional isolation.

130. A) Psychostimulants
Psychostimulants are used for first-line treatment of ADHD because they function through blockage and reuptake of dopamine as well as norepinephrine. First- and second-generation antipsychotics are used for treating schizophrenia by lowering the activity of dopamine. Anticonvulsant medications change the electrical conductivity inside the membranes and, therefore, help in treating bipolar disorder.

131. B) Rivastigmine
Alzheimer disease is usually treated with drugs that target acetylcholine or glutamate. Cholinesterase inhibitors are used for treating Alzheimer disease because they function by slowing down the rate of memory loss. Rivastigmine is the cholinesterase inhibitor approved for treating mild to severe Alzheimer disease as well as Parkinson disease because it focuses on the improvement of the function of the brain's nerve cells. Donepezil and galantamine are used only for treating Alzheimer disease. Paraoxon is used in the treatment of Alzheimer disease and can also be used for treating glaucoma.

132. A) Hypothyroidism
Lithium has adverse effects on endocrine function by lowering the secretion of thyroid hormones, potentially causing hypothyroidism. Thrombocytopenia, liver failure, and pancreatitis do not occur as a result of lithium but can occur due to the adverse effects of an anticonvulsant medicine.

133. D) Blurred vision
Lithium is used to manage symptoms of mania in a bipolar patient. Lithium toxicity has symptoms like dry mouth, vomiting, blurred vision, headache, diarrhea, dizziness, and hypothyroidism. It can cause weight gain. Hypotension, rather than hypertension, is another side effect of lithium toxicity. Insomnia is not a side effect of lithium administration.

134. B) Selegiline (Eldepryl)
The only antidepressant medicine available as a transdermal patch is selegiline. Phenelzine, isocarboxazid, and tranylcypromine are MAOIs used for treating depression, but none are available as a patch.

135. C) Insomnia

Ramelteon (Rozerem) is a drug that has been approved by the U.S. Food and Drug Administration to treat insomnia, in which the patient faces difficulty staying asleep. Based on the receptor the drug binds to, it helps with either regulating sleep or regulating the circadian rhythm. Sleep paralysis, anxiety, and paranoia are not official indications for ramelteon.

136. A) Delusions and hallucinations in schizophrenia

The symptoms of schizophrenia occur due to the overactivity of dopamine in the mesolimbic system, which causes hallucinations and delusions. First-generation antipsychotics act as antagonists of dopamine in the central nervous system. They bind to the D2 receptors and decrease the binding of dopamine, which helps in reducing dopaminergic stimulation. This ultimately reduces delusions and hallucinations in patients with schizophrenia. Bipolar disorder is treated with anticonvulsant medication, and insomnia is treated with benzodiazepines, not antipsychotics.

137. B) Mirtazapine (Remeron)

Insomnia can be treated with mirtazapine, which belongs to the category of noradrenergic and serotonergic antidepressants. Bupropion is used for treating sexual dysfunction and fatigue. Fluoxetine is an antidepressant that is not used to treat insomnia. Duloxetine helps in reducing pain.

138. D) Selective serotonin reuptake inhibitors

Selective serotonin reuptake inhibitors such as paroxetine (Paxil) are mostly used as the first line of defense against anxiety disorders. Benzodiazepine compositions are used only after the intensity of anxiety is reduced. Beta-blockers can treat generalized anxiety issues. Serotonin and norepinephrine reuptake inhibitors help in treating severe as well as generalized anxiety disorders, but paroxetine is not one of them.

139. B) Mirtazapine (Remeron)

Mirtazapine acts as a norepinephrine and serotonin-specific antidepressant. Patients with weight loss and severe appetite loss or insomnia often receive this treatment. Mirtazapine binds as an antagonist with the postsynaptic serotonin receptor. Paroxetine is a selective serotonin reuptake inhibitor. Bupropion is a norepinephrine and dopamine reuptake inhibitor. Vortioxetine is a serotonin modulator and stimulant.

140. C) Lithium

Lithium is considered the gold standard among mood stabilizers to treat patients with bipolar disorder. Lithium interacts in a complex manner to stabilize the electrical activity in the neurons. Sodium and potassium directly take part in the process of neurotransmission; hence, they do not affect the patient. Introducing them in excess will only lead to ionic imbalance in the body. Monoamine oxidase degrades neurotransmitters.

141. A) Antipsychotic

Chlorpromazine was the first antipsychotic drug that functioned by blocking the D2 receptors of the postsynaptic neurons in the mesolimbic pathway. Analgesics are painkillers, antipyretic drugs reduce fever, and antispasmodic medications relieve muscle spasms.

142. B) Cholinesterase inhibitors

The use of cholinesterase inhibitors slows down the effects of Alzheimer disease. As the cholinesterase is inhibited, the effect of acetylcholine increases, which inhibits the breakdown of cholinergic neurons. Muscle blockers are used in the process of anesthesia. Antipsychotics reduce and control many psychotic symptoms but do not control degradation due to Alzheimer disease. Lithium acts as a mood stabilizer, but it does not affect Alzheimer disease because it affects the serotonergic neurons.

143. B) Absorption, distribution, transformation, and removal of a drug from the body

Pharmacokinetics is the study of how a drug is absorbed and distributed in the body. It also studies the transformation of the drug for use and how it is excreted from the body. Pharmacodynamics is the study of the effect of a drug on the body. Pharmacogenetics studies the effect of genetic factors in determining a person's metabolic response to a particular drug or medication. Pharmacovigilance is the study of prevention of the adverse effects of medications.

144. A) Attention deficit hyperactivity disorder

Straterra is prescribed for adult and childhood attention deficit hyperactivity disorder. This medication is a preferred choice for people who experience anxiety while taking stimulants, and it can also be used for comorbid anxiety. Medications like haloperidol (Haldol) are used to treat schizophrenia. Lithium has been used to treat severe agitation in bipolar disorder. Duloxetine (Cymbalta) or tricyclic antidepressants are used for treating depression.

145. C) Cognitive behavioral

Cognitive behavioral therapy (CBT) acts along with medications to treat depression. Due to the seriousness of the patient's issues, the proper active and challenging therapy is necessary. Family therapy helps the patient and the patient's family to recover from distressing situations. In general, behavioral therapy can treat behavior or anger management problems, but for depression, CBT incorporates additional attention. Behavioral therapy can help the patient to open up, but it is not sufficient for severe depression. Interpersonal therapy is focused on improving the relationships or conflicts in the social or personal life of a patient; it is suitable for interpersonal conflicts.

146. C) Gamma-aminobutyric acid (GABA)

Benzodiazepines like alprazolam have antianxiety and anticonvulsant properties. These bind to the GABA receptor complex, enhance the activity of the neurotransmitter GABA, and produce a calming effect. Serotonin, dopamine, and melatonin are not directly impacted by benzodiazepines.

147. B) Let the patient cry for some time and then discuss the issues after the patient settles

The nurse should give the patient time to cry and should offer empathy. Crying helps suppressed emotions to surface and enables the nurse to communicate with the patient. The nurse should not ask the patient to stop crying because this would suppress the expression of the patient's emotions. The nurse can provide tissues to the patient and wait until the patient feels like speaking again. The nurse should not ask the patient to go outside to cry because this will not help the office provide a safe space for open communication. Hugging or touching a patient depends on several factors. The nurse should usually refrain from physical contact with the patient, as it can cause ethical issues. Hugging a patient is a personal decision; however, generally, it is not an appropriate response to a crying patient.

148. A) Triangulation

Bringing in a third person to resolve conflict is triangulation. Triangulation can occur with a child, parent, sibling, or close friend. Modeling occurs when a person imitates the behavior of another in order to alter their own behavior. A cross-generational coalition occurs when one person makes a coalition with another person from a different generation. The parent–child coalition is an example of such a coalition. A covert coalition occurs when the coalition is not readily apparent. The coalition in the patient's situation is visible and direct; it is not covert.

149. B) Serum thyroid-stimulating hormone

The patient's reported symptoms suggest a thyroid disorder. Serum thyroid-stimulating hormone (TSH) measures the amount of TSH produced by the pituitary gland, which regulates hormones released by the thyroid. It is appropriate to order a medical workup when physical causes are suspected; however, there is no correlation with blood alcohol level, liver function tests, or electrocardiogram changes with the patient's symptoms.

150. B) Olanzapine (Zyprexa)

Olanzapine (Zyprexa) is an atypical antipsychotic. Atypical antipsychotics are known to increase risk factors for metabolic syndrome. The patient's elevated HbA1C, lipid profile, weight gain, and increase in abdominal girth are signs of metabolic syndrome. Citalopram (Celexa) is a selective serotonin reuptake inhibitor (SSRI) and is not known to contribute to metabolic syndrome. Dextroamphetamine (Adderall) is a stimulant; weight loss would be more likely with this medication. Sertraline (Zoloft) is an SSRI with no association with metabolic syndrome.

Printed in the United States
by Baker & Taylor Publisher Services